Bedside
Diagnosis

Bedside Diagnosis

An Annotated Bibliography of Literature on Physical Examination and Interviewing

HENRY SCHNEIDERMAN, MD, FACP

Professor of Medicine (Geriatrics)
and Associate Professor of Pathology,
University of Connecticut School of Medicine,
and Travelers Center on Aging,
Farmington, Connecticut;
Physician-in-Chief, Hebrew Home & Hospital, West Hartford, Connecticut

ALDO J. PEIXOTO, MD

Post-Doctoral Fellow in Nephrology,
Yale University School of Medicine,
New Haven, Connecticut

THIRD EDITION

American College of Physicians
Philadelphia, Pennsylvania

A|C|P

Manager, Book Publishing: David Myers
Acquisitions Editor: Mary K. Ruff
Production Supervisor: Allan S. Kleinberg
Production Editor: Victoria Hoenigke
Cover Designer: Kate Nixon

Third Edition

Copyright © 1997 by American College of Physicians

Printed in the United States of America
Composition by Fulcrum Data Services, Inc.
Printing/binding by Versa Press, Inc.

American College of Physicians
Independence Mall West
Sixth Street at Race
Philadelphia, PA 19106-1572

Library of Congress Cataloging-in-Publication Data

Schneiderman, Henry, 1951-
    Bedside diagnosis: an annotated bibliography of literature on physical examination and interviewing/by Henry Schneiderman and Aldo J. Peixoto.—3rd ed.
    p.   cm.
    Includes indexes.
    ISBN 0-943126-55-X (alk. paper)
    1. Physical diagnosis—Bibliography.   2. Medical history taking—Bibliography.   I. Peixoto, Aldo J.   II. Title.
    [DNLM: 1. Diagnosis—abstracts.   2. Medical History Taking—abstracts.   3. Physical Examination—abstracts.   ZWB 200 S359b 1997]
    Z6664.8.P58S36   1997
    [RC71]
    016.61607′54—dc21
    DNLM/DLC
    for Library of Congress   96-29487
                                                                                    CIP

97 98 99 00 01 02/9 8 7 6 5 4 3 2 1

To the memory of my beloved parents

Moe Schneiderman (1913–1973)
and
Betty Bernstein Schneiderman (1919–1976)

and to the memory of

Hacib Aoun, MD (1955–1992)
a brave friend and respected colleague

H.S.

To my parents

Aldo Jose Peixoto
and
Ana Kotzias Peixoto

ultimate sources of incentive and unconditional love

A.J.P., Filho

Authors' Note

Many clinicians express dissatisfaction with their own bedside diagnostic skills and perceive an atrophy of these skills across the profession. This bibliography is intended to remedy one part of the problem: lack of awareness about, and thus ready access to, sources of helpful information. The widest possible range of sources and useful topics was reviewed in choosing the works cited.

Acknowledgments

My wife, Rosemaria Memoli, offered many constructive, critical insights. She and our son, Joseph Natale Schneiderman, tolerated my working endlessly on this project, inevitably at the expense of our time together. I will always remain grateful to them for this among many other reasons.—*H.S.*

Ms. Joan Radeen tirelessly handled a volume of secretarial work relating to this project that exceeded what should be asked of anybody, and she always did so cheerfully and expertly. Jessica Davidson dug out many obscure articles. Joel Brown jumped in with both feet, most helpfully, at the two-minute warning. We are most grateful to each of these people. Our thanks also to the publications staff of the American College of Physicians, who were consistently professional, practical, supportive, and helpful. This work was completed in part while Dr. Peixoto was Chief Resident in Internal Medicine at the University of Connecticut School of Medicine.—*H.S. and A.J.P.*

Introduction to the Third Edition

Clinicians worldwide continue to produce new work on physical diagnosis that can be employed daily at the bedside, to the great benefit of patients everywhere. The prospect of improving our clinical work—that is, taking better care of the patients, who are the *raison d'être* of medicine—means that an updating and rewriting of *Bedside Diagnosis* was indispensable and timely.

For this edition we have included a great many new papers and books. We have also become much tougher about removing older works. We have rewritten many of the commentaries to make them clearer and more useful. We realize that even the most dedicated physician will be unable to find the time to read every article or book of interest. This being so, readers will rely on our statements and summaries. We have included critical comments because we recognize that these form as important a help to the practicing physician as do favorable comments.

Two other major changes mark this third edition. First, it is no longer a one-author work. Many constructive and collegial disagreements between the two of us have enriched our choices of which papers to include, which to exclude, and what to say about each. Second, we have deleted the author addresses that were a feature of the second edition on grounds of their not being utilized. If the reader *does* wish to contact the author of an article referenced in this book, he or she may write to the published address for reprints; lacking the article in hand to check this, the reader should visit or telephone a medical library that will have national and international listings of physicians. The reader may also search various sources on the Internet.

Many important articles have not been included in this bibliography, and readers are welcome to suggest candidates for a future edition. No one can know every good work that is out there, and no two readers will judge the same set of papers to be indispensable. We have tried to avoid articles on imaging, laboratory studies, and other topics that exceed the scope of this work. Physical diagnosis illuminates an immense set of issues for every clinician, but it is only one part of the universe of medicine.

The computer searching of the literature for this edition was performed in mid-1996; the most recent article included herein dates from that year.

Henry Schneiderman, MD, FACP
Aldo J. Peixoto, MD

Introduction to the First Edition (in part)

The large amount of literature on bedside diagnosis continues to grow. Most practitioners, trainees, and teachers remain unaware of this literature and do not go beyond introductory textbooks to address questions on physical diagnosis. This bibliography was compiled to extend the resources of physicians.

A computerized search of the medical literature from 1974 through 1984 was done using standard descriptors for interviewing and examination. From among 4000 citations (a third of which proved relevant), those sources with the most new information and applicability, highest quality science, and most lucid presentation were selected. Monthly update searches, using the same descriptors, added citations through 1987. Materials not retrieved in the search, literature for which key (indexing) terms did not reflect its significant content on bedside diagnosis, materials collected by the author and by others, and references cited throughout the medical literature were also reviewed.

In selecting entries, accessibility for physicians was considered. If a journal cited here is not available, a reference librarian (and very likely use of Inter-Library Loan) can help locate it. Many authors also have large supplies of reprints, particularly if their article appeared in a lesser-known journal.

Contents

General Material

1. **Fitzgerald FT. The clinical examination: a dying art?** *Forum on Medicine*. **1980;May:348-9.**

   Passionate, insightful, and entertaining plea to restore the primacy of the bedside interview and examination.

2. **Frank CW. Gift at Bar Mitzvah.** *Ann Intern Med*. **1993;119:1049.**

   The perspective of a father giving his son a stethoscope as entree to the profession, speculating on its use for connecting with patients, and reminding the listener that the purpose of it all is to "improve our effectiveness in caring for patients." Beautifully said.

3. **Frank SH, Stange KC, Moore P, Smith CK. The focused physical examination: should checkups be tailor-made?** *Postgrad Med*. **1992;92(2):171-86.**

   Looks at the United States Preventive Services Task Force recommendations, among others, and considers individualized alternatives. Thoughtful explication on the nondiagnostic advantages of examining patients, and, equally valuable, on the downside of over-doing the examination or of overemphasizing it.

4. Frame PS. The complete annual physical examination refuses to die [Editorial]. *J Fam Pract*. 1995;40:543-5.

   A wise and articulate statement by one of the early experts in selectivity, tailored to those conditions in which there is scientific evidence that intervention and early diagnosis improve outcome. Delineates how complete physical examination and complete patient evaluation differ. Practical and *not* heartless as are so many discussions in this domain.

5. **Hardison JE. Observations on selected physical findings.** *Emory Univ J Med*. **1988;2:205-17.**

   A fine collection of signs, some never published before, reflecting long, intense, and informed study by a master examiner.

6. **Hardison JE. "The sky is falling."** *Am J Med*. **1980;68:163.**

   A set of very funny, insightful comments that remains enjoyable 17 years and many readings later.

7. **Kampmeier RH. The physical examination: an art [Editorial].** *South Med J.* **1988;81:687-90.**

    Insights from a distinguished physician whose textbook of physical diagnosis was already in its final edition in 1970.

8. **Kampmeier RH. Medicine as an art: the history and physical examination.** *South Med J.* **1982;75:203-10.**

    Marvelous reflection, using the most cogent examples from the history of medicine.

9. **Longson D. The clinical consultation.** *J R Coll Phys Lond.* **1983;17:192-5.**

    How we garner information and make and test hypotheses at the bedside. A "metaphysics of interview and examination." Describes the *nature*, not the detail, of the examiner's task. Advocates a biopsychosocial approach without using that term.

10. **Nardone DA, Lucas LM, Palac DM. Physical examination: a revered skill under scrutiny.** *South Med J.* **1988;81:770-3.**

    The place of the modality today, and a statement of the "challenge for tomorrow . . . to determine the operating characteristics of physical examination techniques and the clinical utility of physical findings."
    See also a related essay:

11. Nardone DA. The framework of pathognomonic physical findings. *Hosp Pract.* 1990;25(2):72-6.
    In the 19th century, many conditions were defined by their physical findings, corroborated by pathologic specimens. Such a framework does not apply well today, certainly not without modulation.

12. **Peterson MC, Holbrook JH, Hales DV, et al. Contributions of the history, physical examination, and laboratory investigation in making medical diagnoses.** *West J Med.* **1992;156(2):163-5.**

    Most recent re-examination reaffirms, in a practice of four faculty general internists, that 76% of ultimately validated new diagnoses are made during the history, 12% during the physical examination, and 11% from laboratory or imaging studies. Certainty of diagnosis rises commensurately during stepwise assessment.

13. **Sackett DL. A primer on the precision and accuracy of the clinical examination. (The Rational Clinical Examination.)** *JAMA.* **1992;267:2638-44.**

    Insightful article on the uses of epidemiologic theory in clinical examination to assess *accuracy* (correspondence of the finding to the truth) and *precison* (its reproducibility among different clinicians). The content, and Sackett's reputation, make it a "must-read."

14. **Sackett DL. The science of the art of the clinical examination [Editorial].** *JAMA.* **1992;267:2650-2.**

Brief essay on the uses of the clinical examination in medicine and on the limitations of research methodology in the field.

15. **Schneiderman H. Expert selectivity in physical diagnosis [Editorial].** *Consultant.* **1991;31:3.**

Prototype of focused examination in place of the old shibboleth of the complete examination.

16. **Van Peenen HJ. Kipp.** *Ann Intern Med.* **1994;120:1041-2.**

A story that will be familiar, in one form or another, to all clinicians: the sense of inappropriateness and ineptitude with examination skills early in the medical career, and then an important relationship with a stranger who let us learn to be better examiners.

17. **Wiener S, Nathanson M. Physical examination: frequently observed errors.** *JAMA.* **1976;236:852-5.**

Data show how physical examination skills have withered among internists. The authors subclassify errors into such sensible categories as poor ordering and organization of the examination; defective equipment; failure to perform part of the examination; missing a sign that is present; reporting detection of a sign that is not present (see reference 445); and forgetting a finding that has been elicited and not recording it, among several others. They also present promising remedies that require much faculty time.
Related items:

18. Johnson JE, Carpenter JL. Medical house staff performance in physical examination. *Arch Intern Med.* 1986;146:937-41.

More work that has deepened our understanding of the present state of physical examination skills among internists.

19. Wray NP, Friedland JA. Detection and correction of house staff error in physical diagnosis. *JAMA.* 1983;249:1035-7.

Approaches to discovering bad house officer examinations, and to improving them.

Methods of physical examination

20. **Abella M, Formolo J, Penney DG. Comparison of the acoustic properties of six popular stethoscopes.** *J Acoust Soc Am.* **1992;91:2224-8.**

Using an interesting technique, it was shown that low-frequency sounds are amplified by all bells and by the Littmann diaphragms. High-frequency sounds were attenuated by all bells and diaphragms (the corrugated Tycos especially). Despite the good science, one of the authors will continue to use the corrugated diaphragm because of personal experience that it permits detection of many sounds inaudible with, or unclear by using, the other heads.

21. **Bloch H. The fathers of percussion.** *J Fam Pract.* **1993;36:232.**

A reflection on the unreceptive initial response of the medical community to Auenbrugger's *Inventum novum*, in which he described the method of percussion. Concludes with a potent speculation about what other good ideas are presently under ridicule, only to be vindicated by their ultimate use.

22. **Hamlet S, Penney DG, Formolo J. Stethoscope acoustics and cervical auscultation of swallowing.** *Dysphagia.* **1994;9:63-8.**

According to these authors, the best ones to use in dysphagia assessment appear to be the Littmann Cardiology II, and the Hewlett-Packard Rappaport-Sprague with medium bell and small diaphragm. Apparently mistakenly regards the ribbed diaphragm on the Tycos Harvey Triple Head as intended to capture high-frequency rather than low-frequency sound, leading to testing it for the wrong characteristics.

23. **Hayden GF. Olfactory diagnosis in medicine.** *Postgrad Med.* **1980; 67:110-8.**

Compilation of smells that assist diagnosis. Tables separate urinary odors from those of the skin, breath, and so on.

24. **Karr MD. Just reach out and percuss someone [Letter].** *JAMA.* **1992; 268:604.**

Demonstrates that auscultation can be attempted through an ordinary telephone, with the mouthpiece at the other end held to the patient's chest. Karr found unreported wheezes in this manner. The title, a reworking of a jingle for the telephone company, is inaccurate.

25. **McGee SR. Percussion and physical diagnosis: separating myth from science.** *Dis Mon.* **1995;41:641-92.**

Exhaustive analysis of the literature on percussion in physical diagnosis. The detail of discussion, with a solid historical perspective and citation of 163 references, makes this monograph the most authoritative on the subject. The author discusses the evidence to substantiate the use of percussion in practice and concludes in favor of its use in only three instances: detection of pleural effusions, evaluation of ascites by the method of shifting dullness, and auscultatory percussion of the shoulder. Despite McGee's refuting other uses of percussion, we still believe the literature gives adequate support for its use in the evaluation of cardiac, hepatic, and splenic size when combined with other bedside techniques.

26. Sapira JD . . . . And how big is the spleen? *South Med J.* 1981;74:53-62.

A closely reasoned and passionate argument about being scientific in medical diagnosis and about the inconsistency of recording liver span by percussion while refusing to accept the validity of percussing cardiac borders.

27. **Orton D, Stryker R. Sick stethoscope syndrome [Letter].** *JAMA.* **1986;256:2817.**

Despite the arch presentation, one valid point can be found in this letter: inattention to the condition of diagnostic instruments presents the hazard of erroneous findings and improper conclusions, leading to futile work-up.

28. Ciferri F. Sick stethoscopes modified and debugged [Letter]. *JAMA.* 1987;257:1331-2.

This letter is priggish but makes a point: Proper sequence of examination helps avert problems of false sounds created as artefacts. It might be added that defective equipment makes trouble even for the perfect examiner and therefore needs to be recognized and fixed right away.

29. **Schneiderman H. Do attending physicians really percuss?** *Am J Med.* **1991;91:325-7.**

Editorial accompanying the Heckerling paper (*see* reference 360). Provides a historical context for cardiac percussion and a consideration of its place today.

30. **Watkinson JC, Johnston D, Jones N, et al. The reliability of palpation in the assessment of tumours.** *Clin Otolaryngol.* **1990;15:405-9.**

Animal model used, with comparison of persons at different levels of training. Considers sources of false-positive and false-negative results. Applicability to humans remains to be determined.

Reference standards

31. **Naylor CD, McCormack DG, Sullivan SN. The midclavicular line: a wandering landmark.** *Can Med Assoc J.* **1987;136:48-50.**

Discusses the problem with assumptions and measurements based on this seemingly unmistakable anatomic site. The situation is worse in the obese, and the variation in site reported by different examiners may be as much as 10 cm!

Screening

32. **Oboler SK, LaForce FM. The periodic physical examination in asymptomatic adults.** *Ann Intern Med.* **1989;110:214-26.**

This article has been unjustly reviled in searing correspondence. The authors acknowledge that the physical examination serves many functions above and beyond diagnosis. They also note that its role in the presence of symptoms differs vastly from its role in screening. The review provides a short list of maneuvers for which there is rigorous evidence of reduced morbidity or mortality. The suggestions for rethinking routine physicals are gentle, rational, and nonderogatory.

33. **United States Public Health Service. Cancer detection in adults by physical examination.** *Am Fam Phys.* **1995;51:871-4, 877-80, 883-5.**

Consideration of the United States Preventive Services Task Force and several other sets of screening guidelines. Detailed advice on using examinations of the breasts, mouth, skin, thyroid, and rectum, as well as, separately, genitalia in both sexes.

Technology and physical diagnosis

34. **Adolph RJ. The value of bedside examination in an era of high technology—Part I.** *Heart Dis Stroke.* **1994;3(3):128-31.**

An established authority on auscultation (*see* reference 377) wisely advises the reader to mimic heart sounds and murmurs as a means of characterizing and understanding them. Explains why audibility of S2 at the apex does not exclude mitral regurgitation. However, criteria for deciding which ejection murmurs require echocardiography in search of aortic stenosis miss the insights of reference 390.

35. **Calin A, Porta J, Fries JF, Schurman DJ. Clinical history as a screening test for ankylosing spondylitis.** *JAMA.* **1977;237:2613-4.**

Shows that the predictive value of a positive test—using five questions about insidious onset before the age of 40 years, persistence for longer than 3 months, morning stiffness, and improvement with exercise—appears to be as high as that of the expensive human lymphocyte antigen (HLA) typing. A marvelous use of sense and insight.

36. **Carter J, Fowler J, Carson L, et al. How accurate is the pelvic examination compared with transvaginal sonography? A prospective, comparative study.** *J Reprod Med.* **1994;39(1):32-4.**

Significant discordance exists between the two methods in a study conducted at a women's cancer center, with frequent underestimation of ovarian size being the most troublesome single deficit of bimanual examination, along with labeling as a mass sonographically undetectable tissue. The technologic method also has imperfect concordance with subsequent laparoscopic findings. The authors carefully note that bimanual examination should not be abandoned and that examiner experience, patient weight, and degree of muscular relaxation bear on efficacy of bimanual palpation, which corresponded perfectly to sonography more than three fourths of the time.

37. **Filly RA. Ultrasound: the stethoscope of the future, alas.** *Radiology.* **1988;167:400.**

What makes for a bad bedside physical examiner also makes for an inept ultrasonographer. Entertaining and valid.

38. **Fitzgerald FT. Physical diagnosis versus modern technology: a review.** *West J Med.* **1990;152:377-82.**

A consideration of the relative power of the two. Written in a spirit that means to open rather than close the discussion of the functions and values of bedside evaluation for the future. Serves as a response to Nardone's plea (*see* reference 10).

39. **Forker AD. The lost art of physical diagnosis [Editorial].** *Hosp Pract (Off Ed).* **1994;29(3):11-2.**

According to the author, "Not every patient with a systolic murmur needs an echocardiogram," and the answer to any query about a murmur is not "I am waiting for the echo report." See reference 40 for supportive data.

40. **Grayburn PA, Smith MD, Handshoe R, et al. Detection of aortic insufficiency by standard echocardiography, pulsed Doppler echocardiography, and auscultation.** *Ann Intern Med.* **1986;104:599-605.**

Shows that auscultation outperforms standard echocardiography but not pulsed Doppler study. One must pick the correct test if one is to learn more than can be shown by the physical examination; the blind choice of "echo" clearly will not serve.

41. **LaCombe MA. The cabalist.** *JAMA.* **1988;259:3045.**

A most entertaining projection into a future (or present?) in which a medical student who learns the physical signs of aortic insufficiency is regarded as mystical and suspect.

42. **Petty TL. The forgotten vital signs.** *Hosp Pract (Off Ed).* **1994;29:11-2.**

Advocates elevating the hand-held spirometer from technologic investigation to bedside tool of every physician. Cogently presents the historical analogy of the role of the sphygmomanometer.

43. **Riegelman RK. The dogged physical examination in the era of the CAT.** *Prim Care.* **1980;7:625-35.**

A refreshing review of the rationales for, and benefits and limitations of, various components of physical examination. Employs the imaginative and useful viewpoint that physical examination is a new technology whose adoption must be justified.

Textbooks of physical examination

44. **Bates B, Bickley LS, Hoekelman RA.** *A Guide to Physical Examination and History Taking.* **6th ed. Philadelphia: JB Lippincott; 1995.**

    Popular but simplistic and very short on pathophysiology.

45. **DeGowin RL.** *DeGowin & DeGowin's Diagnostic Examination.* **6th ed. New York: McGraw-Hill, Inc.; 1994.**

    A pocket guide that, because it now exceeds 1000 pages, has outgrown its portability. The book would benefit immensely from a weeding out of the portions that are now outdated and from revisiting the illustrations, once charmingly naive and now merely uninformative.

46. **Epstein O, Perkin GD, de Bono DP, Cookson J.** *Clinical Examination.* **St. Louis: Mosby–Year Book; 1992.**

    Lavishly and very well illustrated. Packed with information. Rather idiosyncratic proportioning, so that, as with most textbooks in this area, it does not supersede a textbook of medicine.

47. **Sapira JD.** *The Art and Science of Bedside Diagnosis.* **Baltimore: Urban & Schwarzenberg; 1990.**

    A splendid work of great depth, by a critical and iconoclastic thinker who knows the field intimately from long practice and intense scholarship. Not a book for beginners but an unparalleled joy for the seasoned teacher or practitioner.

48. **Walker HK, Hall WD, Hurst JW, eds.** *Clinical Methods.* **3rd ed. Boston: Butterworths; 1990.**

    One symptom, examination technique, sign, or laboratory finding is presented at a time, in each of the numerous, exceptionally brief chapters. Particularly helpful for focused learning by the established clinician oriented to bedside evaluation.

49. **Willms JL, Schneiderman H, Algranati PS.** *Physical Diagnosis: Bedside Evaluation of Diagnosis and Function.* **Baltimore: Williams & Wilkins; 1994.**

    Addresses the separate needs of the beginning student and the more experienced clinician by providing a basic examination for each body region, and then a more advanced section for each region, incorporating problem-focused subroutines for the more expert examiner.

50. **Zitelli BJ, Davis HW.** *Atlas of Pediatric Physical Diagnosis.* **2nd ed. London: Wolfe Publishing; 1993.**

A superbly written and illustrated compendium of signs in children. The quality of the abundant photographs exceeds that of all other books in physical diagnosis and sets a standard while providing accessible, authoritative information for the practitioner.

Interviewing and History-Taking

General material

51. **Bellet PS, Maloney MJ. The importance of empathy as an interviewing skill in medicine.** *JAMA.* **1991;266:1831-2.**

    Describes the cost-effectiveness of empathy, among other points, and the delineation of the difference between empathy, reassurance, and patient education.

52. **Blau JN. Time to let the patient speak.** *Br Med J.* **1989;298:39.**

    This study shows that the much-touted "uninterrupted narrative of the patient" averages less than 2 minutes. Beyond the strict time constraints set by universal busyness, every doctor needs to keep working on promoting "openness" while fortifying the means to rein in gabby patients nondestructively.

53. **Branch WT. The language of patient care.** *J Gen Intern Med.* **1989;4:359.**

    Jargon, ordinary language, and the choice of phrases that relate to the experience and the world of the patient are discussed. This exposition begins as a comment on a study and ends with a most pertinent suggestion.

54. **Brown JB, Weston WW, Stewart MA. Patient-centered interviewing. Part II: Finding common ground.** *Can Fam Physician.* **1989;35:153-7.**

    An understanding of patients' perspectives and of their importance in case management plans forms the proper focus of the search for common ground between patient and clinician.
    Related and useful adjacent papers:

55. Stewart MA, Brown JB, Weston WW. Patient-centered interviewing. Part III: Five provocative questions. *Can Fam Physician.* 1989;35:159-61.

    A review of the effectiveness of patient-centered interviewing in improving patient satisfaction and compliance, concluding in its favor. One shortcoming is the limited methodologic insight and detail.

56. Weston WW, Brown JB, Stewart MA. Patient-centered interviewing. Part I: Understanding patients' experiences. *Can Fam Physician.* 1989;35:147-51.

    Discusses how focusing the history on the patient, not on disease processes, improves the quality and outcome of the patient-physician relationship. Special concerns include the patient's ideas and feelings about the illness, the impact of the illness on function, and patient's expectations of the doctor during the interaction. Practical applicability still seems difficult in the busy context of practice, notwithstanding the answer given to the question of time in the third paper of this series. The conference summary is particularly worthwhile if one lacks access to the other papers (references 54-56).

57. Simpson M, Buckman R, Stewart M, et al. Doctor-patient communication: the Toronto consensus statement. *BMJ.* 1991;303:1385-7.

Consensus of a panel of experts on patient-physician relationship. A concise, well-referenced review of recognized communication problems between the two parties. Several questions are posed as how to best address these deficits from both psychosocial and educational perspectives.

58. **Cassell EJ. *Talking with Patients* (2 volumes). Cambridge, MA: MIT Press; 1985.**

Extensive transcripts of interviews. Provides more insight and good advice than any other source.

59. **Doyle E. A little-taught skill: using the telephone as a medical instrument. *ACP Observer.* 1993;13(2):4.**

Informal description of effective techniques of telephone interviewing and counseling. Body language and other clues are lost. Use of directive questions is important, as are providing reassurance and establishing parameters for follow-up calls. Reiterates the difficulty of third-party interviews and acknowledges both the difficulties of this mode and that patients have expectations for something other than a diagnosis and attendant choice of treatment.

60. **Hardison JE. Whatever happened to the chief complaint? *JAMA.* 1981;245:1942.**

Why writing "Admitted for chemotherapy" as the chief complaint shortchanges the patient.

61. **Herzog A. Thoughts about listening. *Conn Med.* 1991;55:585-6.**

Discusses listening to the patient's words, the messages between the lines, one's family, and oneself.

62. **Kassirer JP, Kopelman RI. The accuracy of clinical information. I: The history. *Hosp Pract.* 1991;26(4):21-4, 29-30.**

Brief discussion of accuracy, validity, and reliability of the medical history. Clinical vignettes are presented to illustrate strategies for improving these attributes. The authors are well known for their book on clinical reasoning and for their regular column on this topic in the *New England Journal of Medicine.*

63. **Lichtenstein MJ, Schaffner W. Assessing activities of daily living [Editorial].** *Hosp Pract.* **1985;20(May 30):8-9.**

Considers the effect of age or any ailment, debility, or disability on a patient's functional status. Such inquiry deserves wider routine use.

64. **Nardone DA, Johnson GK, Faryna A, et al. A model for the diagnostic medical interview: nonverbal, verbal, and cognitive assessments.** *J Gen Intern Med.* **1992;7:437-42.**

Well-written framework for the diagnostic interview. Emphasizes the importance of nonverbal cues, verbal skills, and the need for critical focus toward diagnostic reasoning.

65. **Novack DH. Beyond data gathering: twelve functions of the medical history [Editorial].** *Hosp Pract.* **1985;20(3A):11-2.**

Lists these 12 functions, drawing on the Society of General Internal Medicine (SGIM) Medical Interviewing Task Force's core curriculum (*see* reference 866). Some key functions are putting the patient at ease, overcoming barriers to communication, avoiding jargon, formulating and testing diagnostic hypotheses, attending to one's own affective reactions to the patient as diagnostically meaningful data, evaluating family relationships, and providing reassurance.

66. **Platt FW, McMath JC. Clinical hypocompetence: the interview.** *Ann Intern Med.* **1979;91:898-902.**

Brilliant exposition of five syndromes of defective interviewing, namely low therapeutic content, flawed data base, defective hypothesis generation, failure to demand primary data, and inappropriately high-control style. Material on why interviews go wrong and on conversational and interactional styles of various patients is valuable. Every clinician should read this gem annually.

67. Hooper PL, Hooper EM, Stehr DE. Guidelines for interviewing [Letter]. *Ann Intern Med.* 1981;95:238.

Veterans Affairs providers respond to Platt's acute insights. We can immediately treat patients more humanely and, in the process, gather better information. Brief, specific instructions.

Difficult interviews

68. **Coulehan JL. Who is the poor historian?** *JAMA.* **1984;252:221.**

The term describes the interviewer at least as often as the patient to whom the label is being attached: "More time listening to the patient and less . . . agonizing over . . . a magnesium value would be a step in the right direction."

69. **Einterz EM. Cultural barriers and the diagnostic process [Letter].** *Lancet.* **1987;1:1434.**

Astute observations based on experience with the Tiv people of central Nigeria. Concerns the difficulty of translating both language and culture when the reference points and belief systems of physician and patient are separated by an apparently impassable gulf.

70. **Mackenzie TB. The initial patient interview: identifying when psychosocial factors are at work.** *Postgrad Med.* **1983;74:259-65.**

The conversational tone of this article belies well-conceived techniques for recognizing clues that a patient's agenda differs from one's own.

71. **Putsch RW III. Cross-cultural communication: the special case of interpreters in health care.** *JAMA.* **1985;254:3344-8.**

Makes numerous sound observations. The broader topic of dealing with patients from unfamiliar social strata or backgrounds is discussed in Putsch and Marlie Joyce's chapter, "Dealing with Patients from Other Cultures" (pages 1050-65, *see* reference 48 for complete citation).

Occupational history

72. **Occupational and Environmental Health Committee of the American Lung Association of San Diego and Imperial Counties. Taking the occupational history.** *Ann Intern Med.* **1983;99:641-51.**

Clearly stated guidelines. Useful, comprehensible tables and lists. A comprehensive form, designed for patients to record work and exposure histories, is included for photocopying.

Sexual history

73. **Bachmann GA, Leiblum SR, Grill J. Brief sexual inquiry in gynecologic practice.** *Obstet Gynecol.* **1989;73:425-7.**

Discusses how in 887 consecutive women seen in a gynecologic practice, direct inquiry about sexual activity and "sexual difficulties or problems" markedly increased the prevalence of sexual complaints (from 3% to 19%). Shows that simple questioning is effective and well received.

74. **Ende J, Rockwell S, Glasgow M. The sexual history in general medicine practice.** *Arch Intern Med.* **1984;144:558-61.**

This carefully designed study shows that both physicians and patients find *routine* exploration of sexual function valuable.

75. Gremminger RA. Taking a sexual history. *Wis Med J.* 1983;82:20-4.

Focuses on sexually transmitted diseases. Includes "street terms." The explicit discussion of unusual behaviors will render informed physicians less liable to be shocked. Contains some stereotypes.

76. Segraves KA, Segraves RT, Schoenberg HW. Use of sexual history to differentiate organic from psychogenic impotence. *Arch Sex Behav.* 1987;16(2):125-37.

Discusses how in 32 patients with impotence (using nocturnal penile tumescence [NPT] recordings as the gold standard) questions about early morning erections correctly identified 100% of patients with organic causes of impotence (no early morning erections and an abnormal NPT study), and 86% of those with psychogenic erectile dysfunction (normal erection on NPT). Unfortunately, no mention is made of the convenient, low-technology postage-stamp test to help one in the nonresearch setting.

77. Stevenson RW, Szasz G, Maurice WL, Miles JE. How to become comfortable talking about sex to your patients. *Can Med Assoc J.* 1983;128:797-800.

Most useful if read in conjunction with any of the above-mentioned articles.

Social history including substance abuse history

78. Paton A, Saunders JB. ABC of alcohol: asking the right questions. *Br Med J.* 1981;283:1458-9.

The CAGE and other screening questions, some proven to increase accuracy of detecting alcoholism, can be learned and used with minimal time investment. The limitations of questionnaires and of microcomputer "interviews" are stressed.

79. Westreich LM, Rosenthal RN. Physical examination of substance abusers: how to gather evidence of concealed problems. *Postgrad Med.* 1995;97(4):111-2,117-20,123.

Includes the classic triad of piloerection, rhinorrhea, and lacrimation in opiate withdrawal; marked excoriation in cocaine users; finding forgotten needles at injection sites or downstream from same; and the role of body cavity searches as a special variant of physical examination, requiring legal probable cause and appropriate chaperoning.

Family history

80. Love RR. Genetics and human cancer: family history and common cancers. *Wis Med J.* 1987;86:20-1.

The applicability exceeds the best-known rarities such as Gardner syndrome and retinoblastoma.

81. **Milhorn HT Jr. The genogram: a structured approach to the family history.** *J Miss State Med Assoc.* **1981;22:250-2.**

Presents a simple, useful method for recording interpersonal interactions and life-situation data along with family history. Use of symbols minimizes the interviewer's effort and time and the amount of space used in recording these data.

82. **Williams DR. Family history and the risk of complications in diabetes mellitus [Letter].** *Ann Intern Med.* **1986;105:795.**

Recounts flawed but intriguing evidence that a positive family history in a patient with known diabetes predicts the presence of vascular complications.

Values history

83. **Doukas DJ, McCullough LB. The values history: the evaluation of patient's values and advance directives.** *J Fam Pract.* **1991;32:145-53.**

Shows that it is extremely worthwhile to address advance directives routinely rather than in reaction to crisis. The benefits of this approach include avoidance of overtreatment by default.

Review of systems

84. **Hoffbrand BI. Away with the system review: a plea for parsimony.** *Br Med J.* **1989;298:817-9.**

Convincingly argues that a scatter-shot approach is no more productive here than in excessive and nondirected laboratory test ordering.

85. **Mitchell TL, Tornelli JL, Fisher TD, et al. Yield of the screening review of systems: a study on a general medical service.** *J Gen Intern Med.* **1992;7:393-7.**

Employs careful methods and an important approach to the issue, intentionally confined to four cardiorespiratory questions and eight digestive system questions for persons with no prior evidence of problems in these organ systems. Asking about hematochezia may save lives, particularly when the fecal occult-blood test has been negative.

Specific symptoms and syndromes

86. **Atkinson K, Austin DE, McElwain TJ, Peckham MJ. Alcohol pain in Hodgkin's disease.** *Cancer.* **1976;37:895-9.**

Some other neoplasms have also produced pain at sites of primary or metastatic tumor (perhaps via alcohol-mediated vasodilation). The symptom is often misconstrued as psychosomatic until the diagnosis of cancer is made.

87. **Avorn J, Everitt DE, Baker MW. The neglected medical history and therapeutic choices for abdominal pain: a nationwide study of 799 physicians and nurses.** *Arch Intern Med.* **1991;151:694-8.**

In a survey, physicians and nurses responded to a case presentation featuring prominent dyspepsia with discouragingly infrequent requests for the relevant medication history (nonsteroidal anti-inflammatory drugs [NSAIDs] and aspirin). To the extent that this reflects clinical practice, this study shows that even the most pertinent and obvious questions are omitted shockingly often.

88. **Barbezat GO. The vomiting patient: a rational approach.** *Drugs.* **1981;22:246-53.**

Offers powerful, broad-based, and probing questions, based on pathophysiology and differential diagnosis.

89. **Cohen R, Muzaffar S, Capellan J, et al. The validity of classic symptoms and chest radiographic configuration in predicting pulmonary tuberculosis.** *Chest.* **1996;109:420-3.**

Discusses the problem of allocating scarce isolation rooms wisely. Absence of a 2-week-or-longer history of productive cough and weight loss, *combined with* a radiograph atypical for tuberculosis, had a major negative predictive value. The authors discuss why neither symptoms alone nor radiograph alone did the job. Conducted in a group with an extremely high rate of tuberculosis; extrapolation to other groups may be dangerous.

90. **Louria DB, Sen P, Kapila R, et al. Anterior thigh pain or tenderness: a diagnostically useful manifestation of bacteremia.** *Arch Intern Med.* **1985;145:657-8.**

This condition is distinct from ordinary, infectious disease–associated, generalized myalgia.

Physical Examination: General

General appearance

91. **Anonymous. The matchbox sign [Leading article].** *Lancet.* **1983;2:261.**

    How patients with delusions of arthropod infestation often present to the physician carrying a little box in which alleged infesting organisms have been collected, sometimes consisting of recognizably impossible material; legitimately infested persons with the same box in hand should reveal real parasites within it.

92. Lee WR. Matchbox sign [Letter]. *Lancet.* 1983;2:457-8.

    Discusses a variant of the above-mentioned sign. Discusses a patient who brought a small bottle containing metal fragments that she claimed were still being recovered from her nasal mucus, skin eruption, and axillae, 3 years after she had left a workplace of alleged occupational exposure.

93. **Berk SL, Verghese A. General appearance. In: Walker HK, Hall WD, Hurst JW, eds.** *Clinical Methods.* **3rd ed. Boston: Butterworths; 1990:987-9.**

    Well-constructed, brief discussion of how one looks and what one discovers from this type of analysis. Also worthwhile as an entree to the riches of the textbook in which it is located (*see* reference 48).

94. **Dukes RJ. Office evaluation of the pulmonary patient (part I).** *J Indiana State Med Assoc.* **1982;75:794-6.**

    The paragraphs on general appearance and on extrapulmonary signs related to pulmonary diagnoses are excellent. Includes a concise listing of features in the history and examination, including general examination, that lead the clinician to pulmonary diagnoses.

95. **Fitzgerald FT, Tierney LM Jr. The bedside Sherlock Holmes.** *West J Med.* **1982;137:169-75.**

    A wonderful, systematic collection of nonstandard clues derived from the patient, the environs, and the patient's possessions (for example, the wear of the shoes, color of urine stains, and body odors). Emphasizes the utility and pleasure of sharp observation.

96. **Gjørup T, Hendriksen C, Bugge PM, Jensen AM. Global assessment of patients: a bedside study. Part I: The influence of physical findings on the global assessment.** *J Intern Med.* **1989;226:123-5.**

Brave attempt to forge new ground. Realms of agreement and disagreement among observers are striking and not predictable.

97. **Howard RJ, Valori RM. Hospital patients who wear tinted spectacles: physical sign of psychoneurosis. A controlled study.** *J R Soc Med.* **1989; 82:606-8.**

The preconception that "shades" must mean "strange" is not borne out when scrutinized closely.

98. **Kaplan AI, Sabin S. The lipstick sign [Letter].** *Ann Intern Med.* **1981;94:137.**

Describes how a woman who applies lipstick after not wearing it earlier during hospitalization is likely to report feeling subjectively far better as a precondition and may have begun to recover from an acute illness. One of the authors has seen it correlate frequently in women older than 70 years of age, in particular.

99. **Martin L, Khalil H. How much reduced hemoglobin is necessary to generate central cyanosis?** *Chest.* **1990;97:182-5.**

A beautiful and scholarly correction of a prevalent misconception. Reviews the 70-year-old Van Slyke data showing that 5 g/dL of reduced *capillary* hemoglobin is necessary to produce cyanosis in an individual with an average complexion—*not* 5 g of reduced *arterial* blood hemoglobin. In fact, to produce 5 g of deoxygenated arterial blood hemoglobin, the patient would need to be much more hypoxemic. The quantity of desoxyhemoglobin in the capillaries is easy to square with pulse oximetry and cannot be calculated from arterial blood gas values.

100. **Meissner H-H, Franklin C. Extreme hypercapnia in a fully alert patient.** *Chest.* **1992;102:1298-9.**

Reports a patient with chronic obstructive pulmonary disease in acute flare-up who had two arterial P_{CO_2} measurements of more than 100 mm Hg while able to communicate lucidly. This raises questions about the validity of assuming that an unclouded consciousness excludes marked hypercarbia.

101. **Muchmore EA, Dahl BJ. One blue man with mucositis [Letter].** *N Engl J Med.* **1992;327:133.**

Report of methemoglobinemia due to overuse of an over-the-counter topical oral anesthetic in a patient whose widespread stomatitis permitted excess systemic absorption.

102. **Schriger DL, Baraff L. Defining normal capillary refill: variation with age, sex, and temperature.** *Ann Emerg Med.* **1988;17:932-5.**

Reports how capillary refill time was influenced by sex, age, and ambient temperature. Ninety-fifth percentiles for capillary refill time were established in essentially healthy subjects to refute the old "2-second rule." New upper limits of normal for capillary refill that are proposed in this paper are 2 seconds in children and men, 3 seconds in women, and 4 seconds in the elderly. Unfortunately, the study does not augment current spotty, unconvincing knowledge of how to use capillary refill in the assessment of circulatory status.

103. **Sherertz EF, Hess SP. Stated age [Letter].** *N Engl J Med.* **1993;329:281-2.**

Describes the estimation of age of healthy adults based on facial and hand photographs. Tobacco use, fair skin, inadequate solar protection, and frequent alcohol use were associated with older appearance. The guesses of age are alleged to be insufficiently reliable. Failure to cite the work of Model (reference 211), as well as the use of photographs—not a satisfactory proxy for direct inspection—renders this study suspect.

104. **Verghese A. The "typhoid state" revisited.** *Am J Med.* **1985;79:370-2.**

The author is a unique polymath. His literary interest and talent inform a particularly striking exploration of a term that was once familiar and has now returned with regard to patients with late-stage HIV-complication–associated delirium.

Nutritional assessment

105. **Detsky AS, McLaughlin JR, Baker JP, et al. What is subjective global assessment of nutritional status?** *J Parenteral Enteral Nutr.* **1987;11:8-13.**

Detailed description of a method combining history and examination that has been favorably validated against laboratory measures.

106. **Morley JE. Why do physicians fail to recognize and treat malnutrition in older persons?** *J Am Geriatr Soc.* **1991;39:1139-40.**

Includes laboratory and bedside elements but also offers mnemonics to help identify those at risk and those who may have treatable causes of weight loss.

Assessment of volume status

107. **Baraff LJ, Schriger DL. Orthostatic vital signs: variation with age, specificity, and sensitivity in detecting a 450-ml blood loss.** *J Emerg Med.* **1992;10:99-103.**

A discussion of how no combined criteria for orthostatic hypotension/orthostatic tachycardia are sensitive enough to detect intravascular volume depletion in healthy adults who have just donated one unit of blood. The study has significant methodologic limitations.

108. **Eaton D, Bannister P, Mulley GP, Connolly MJ. Axillary sweating in clinical assessment of dehydration in ill elderly patients.** *BMJ.* **1994; 308:1271.**

The characteristics of the test, as reported, do not satisfactorily discriminate between persons with intravascular volume depletion and those without. This important but flawed study needs extension as well as correlation with other clinical indicators such as an increase in resting pulse rate or orthostatic hypotension/orthostatic tachycardia.

109. **Gross CR, Lindquist RD, Woolley AC, et al. Clinical indicators of dehydration severity in elderly patients.** *J Emerg Med.* **1992;10:267-74.**

Describes how mucosal dryness, upper limb weakness, and abnormal sensorium correlate with dehydration. A labor-intensive article that becomes less compelling because of unwarranted statistical techniques to analyze the data. It would have been more useful to determine the predictive value of each clinical variable to estimate severity of dehydration. A good example of the difficulties with methodology in physical diagnosis research.

110. **Koziol-McLain J, Lowenstein SR, Fuller B. Orthostatic vital signs in emergency department patients.** *Ann Emerg Med.* **1991;20:606-10.**

Data were measured with an instrument in patients, primarily young, admitted consecutively to an emergency department. There was a wide variation in persons selected for having no history of blood loss or volume depletion. The average increase in heart rate was 17 bpm, and many of the patients met criteria for orthostatic hypotension, although these did not correspond to those who felt dizziness or thirst. Although much more work is needed, the point is well taken that the range of normal may be wider than previously published norms.

111. Lopez BL. Orthostatic vital signs [Letter]. *Ann Emerg Med.* 1992;21:228-9.

Lists the problems in making sense of orthostatic changes, chief among them being the lack of a gold standard for detecting intravascular volume depletion. Questions the *reliability* of a dip in the diastolic blood pressure, whereas it is the *validity* of this measurement that is inadequate.

112. Schriger DL, Baraff LJ. Capillary refill: is it a useful predictor of hypovolemic states? *Ann Emerg Med.* **1991;20:601-5.**

Study of normal blood donors who have been transiently rendered hypovolemic by donating blood and of emergency department patients with demonstrated orthostatic hypotension or frank hypotension. It is as important to discard unhelpful signs as it is to gain expertise with useful signs.

Vital Signs

Temperature

113. **Azzimondi G, Bassein L, Nonino F, et al. Fever in acute stroke worsens prognosis: a prospective study.** *Stroke.* **1995;26:2040-3.**

    In this study, a temperature greater than 37.9 °C in the first week post-stroke was associated with a threefold increase in the 30-day mortality rate. The major shortcoming of this study is that other underlying causes of fever and their potential impact on mortality are deliberately ignored.

114. **Castle SC, Norman DC, Yeh M, et al. Fever response in elderly nursing home residents: are the older truly colder?** *J Am Geriatr Soc.* **1991;39:853-7.**

    In this study, the mean baseline oral temperature of nursing home patients was lower than published norms (including Mackowiak's norms in younger persons, reference 119). Some elderly patients with "atypically afebrile" infections actually showed an appropriate, "diagnostic" step-up from their subnormal basal temperature.

115. **Ehrenkranz JR. A new method for measuring body temperature.** *N J Med.* **1986;83:93-6.**

    Describes how body temperature is measured through the use of little plastic strips on which the patient voids; a color scale permits reading the result at leisure. This method is convenient for use with small, continent children, with demented persons who reject the thermometer, and in settings in which factitious fever is suspected (*see* reference 831).

116. **Faculty, East of Ireland. How good are we at guessing fever?** *Ir Med J.* **1986;79(1):15-6.**

    The alleged conclusion, that we are *not* very good, is based on observations of severely vitiated methodology including, astoundingly, failing to leave in the thermometer long enough to produce a satisfactory reading!

117. Jolin SW, Howell JM, Milzman DP, et al. **Infrared emission detection tympanic thermometry may be useful in diagnosing acute otitis media.** *Am J Emerg Med.* **1995;13:6-8.**

Describes how the inflamed ear is a little bit warmer than the other ear when the tympanic thermometer is used for bilateral measurements. Cautions about not overinterpreting this but makes the sound point, devising a nomogram, that in the borderline case it may assist decision making.

118. Kiesow LA, Hurley CM. **Fogging in infrared tympanic and ear thermometry [Letter].** *Ann Intern Med.* **1995;122:634-5.**

Describes how keeping the probe within the external auditory canal for 3 minutes induces a rapid and time-dependent decrease in the infrared signal, with progressive lowering of the temperature reading.

119. Mackowiak PA, Wasserman SS, Levine MM. **A critical appraisal of 98.6 degrees Fahrenheit, the upper limit of the normal body temperature, and other legacies of Carl Reinhold August Wunderlich.** *JAMA.* **1992;268:1578-80.**

Shows that the mean oral temperature of healthy young adults on a clinical research unit was 36.8 °C (98.2 °F), not the 37/98.6 popularized by the great 19th century researcher who used 15-minute dwell times in the axilla! Several of his other assertions are strikingly validated.

120. Shinozaki T, Deane R, Perkins F. **Infrared tympanic thermometer: evaluation of a new clinical thermometer.** *Crit Care Med.* **1988;16:148-50.**

Tympanic thermometers showed an excellent correlation ($r = 0.98$) with core measurements in the range of 34 to 39.5 °C.

121. Ogren JM. The inaccuracy of axillary temperatures measured with an electronic thermometer. *Am J Dis Child.* 1990;144:109-11.

One might wish for this fast and less intrusive method to supplant others, but, as this study shows, the site and the instrument combine to vitiate the readings.

122. Tandberg D, Sklar D. **Effect of tachypnea on the estimation of body temperature by an oral thermometer.** *N Engl J Med.* **1983;308:945-6.**

Discusses the way in which tachypnea decreases the measured temperature in a predictable way and may lead to underestimation of fever in patients with acidosis, pulmonary disease, or fever itself, all of which stimulate tachypnea.

123. Watanakunakorn C, Hayek F. **High fever (greater than 39 °C) as a clinical manifestation of pulmonary embolism.** *Postgrad Med J.* **1987;63:951-3.**

Seven cases, all but one in bedbound patients. Important caveat when obscure pulmonary infiltrates or respiratory difficulties are under consideration and one is tempted to discount pulmonary thromboembolic disease on the presumption that high fever excludes noninfectious causes.

Blood pressure

124. **Amar D, Attai LA, Gupta SK, Jones A. Bilateral upper extremity blood pressure measurements should be routine prior to coronary artery surgery [Letter].** *Chest.* **1992;101:882.**

Case report stressing the importance of comparing blood pressure in both upper extremities to screen for subclavian artery stenosis before using left internal mammary artery (LIMA) grafts, lest a subclavian steal syndrome cause myocardial ischemia and infarction.

125. **Amigo I, Cuesta V, Fernandez A, Gonzalez A. The effect of verbal instructions on blood pressure measurement.** *J Hypertension.* **1993;11:293-6.**

Blood pressure fluctuates in the same direction as instructions given regarding the anticipated trend of change, especially the systolic blood pressure.

126. **Bailey RH, Bauer JH. A review of common errors in the indirect measurement of blood pressure: sphygmomanometry.** *Arch Intern Med.* **1993;153:2741-8.**

Thorough, well-referenced review of the topic. A valuable companion to Perloff's American Heart Association guidelines (reference 134).

127. **Belmin J, Visintin J-M, Salvatore R, et al. Osler's maneuver: absence of usefulness for the detection of pseudohypertension in an elderly population.** *Am J Med.* **1995;98:42-9.**

In unselected aged persons, Osler's maneuver was reproducible 90% of the time between two observers, but failed to predict pseudohypertension as judged against the reference standard of intra-arterial manometry.

128. **Cavallini MC, Roman MJ, Blank SG, et al. Association of the auscultatory gap with vascular disease in hypertensive patients.** *Ann Intern Med.* **1996;124:877-83.**

A confusing mixture of high technology and ordinary sphygmomanometry. The central finding appears to be that patients with an audible auscultatory gap—constituting a fifth of persons with hypertension, a number far exceeding our impression of the prevalence of the sign in clinical practice—tend to have more vasculopathy than those without.

129. **Hoffbrand BI. Postexertional hypotension: a valuable physical sign.** *BMJ.* **1982;285:1242.**

Asserts that testing for postexertional decreases in blood pressure may disclose impairment of cardiovascular reflexes, especially sympathetic function. Alleges that when volume depletion is not detected by conventional orthostatic pulse and blood pressure, it can sometimes be found by rechecking the blood pressure after exercise. The cases reported fail to prove this.

130. **Jansen RWMM, Lipsitz LA. Postprandial hypotension: epidemiology, pathophysiology, and clinical management.** *Ann Intern Med.* **1995;122:286-95.**

A detailed review of a notoriously under-recognized problem. Implications for the diagnosis and management of hypertension must be acknowledged: patients all too often come to the office shortly after meals.

131. Peitzman SJ, Berger SR. Postprandial blood pressure decrease in well elderly persons. *Arch Intern Med.* 1989;149:286-8.

Reports that healthy elderly subjects who were not receiving any cardiovascular drugs had a mean decline in blood pressure of 26/13 mm Hg 1 hour after a standard meal. A "water meal" did not reproduce the findings. This is the only such study to find *no* correlation of baseline blood pressure with magnitude of the postprandial drop, perhaps because in these patients no vasoactive drugs were being used.

132. **Messerli FH, Ventura HO, Amodeo C. Osler's maneuver and pseudohypertension.** *N Engl J Med.* **1985;312:1548-51.**

Discusses how an artery that remains palpable distal to a sphygmomanometer inflated enough to occlude the artery suggests that the cuff will overestimate true intra-arterial pressure. The histologic basis of the sign is obscure (*see* reference 437).

133. **Moss AJ. Criteria for diastolic pressure: revolution, counter-revolution, and now a compromise.** *Pediatrics.* **1983;71:854-5.**

Heroically attempts to dissipate murk about Korotkoff sound IV (muffling) versus V (disappearance).

134. **Perloff D, Grim C, Flack J, et al. Human blood pressure determination by sphygmomanometry.** *Circulation.* **1993;88:2460-70.**

Provides explicit instructions, including a particularly useful series of comments on sources of various errors and how to avoid them.

135. **Reeves RA. Does this patient have hypertension? How to measure blood pressure. (The Rational Clinical Examination).** *JAMA.* **1995;273:1211-8.**

Myriad details on technique, significance, improving the diagnosis, and even "the grossest error, not checking BP at all," which "remains a common failing even among cardiovascular specialists." A most useful table (Table 2) starts with the material in the latest AHA guidelines (reference 134) and adds the author's own substantial insights.

136. **Weiss NS. Relation of high blood pressure to headache, epistaxis, and selected other symptoms: the US Health Examination Survey of Adults.** *N Engl J Med.* **1972;287:631-3.**

Large population study showing no relationship between blood pressure, headache, epistaxis, tinnitus, and dizziness. Major flaws of the study are the use of a self-administered questionnaire, unobtainable temporal association between symptoms and blood pressures, and poor detail of questions asked. Although we intended in this text to avoid giving anecdotal commentary, we note that these observations contradict much of our clinical experience.

137. **Zweifler AJ, Shahab ST. Pseudohypertension: a new assessment.** *J Hypertens.* **1993;11:1-6.**

Lucid overview of clinical characteristics of the different types of pseudohypertension. Criteria for diagnosis and useful tips for further investigation are provided.

Orthostatic pulse, blood pressure, and hypotension

138. **Kennedy GT, Crawford MH. Optimal position and timing of blood pressure and heart rate measurements to detect orthostatic changes in patients with ischemic heart disease.** *J Cardiac Rehabil.* **1984;4:219-23.**

Reports that in a model of orthostatic hypotension induced by oral nitrates, use of the sitting position was not adequate to assess postural changes; standing was required. Further reports that blood pressure and pulse should be followed for at least 2 minutes after standing in order to observe and record maximal changes.

139. **Lipsitz LA. Orthostatic hypotension in the elderly.** *N Engl J Med.* **1989;321:952-7.**

A comprehensive review of the subject. Evaluation requires careful technique and close adherence to criteria. Few new therapeutic modalities have emerged since the publication of this classic paper.

140. **Mader SL, Palmer RM, Rubenstein LZ. Effect of timing and number of baseline blood pressure determinations on postural blood pressure response.** *J Am Geriatr Soc.* **1989;37:444-6.**

Shows that supine blood pressure decreases with repeated readings, not with the duration that the patient has lain supine—that is, there is regression to the mean. A single supine reading before standing is fully effective in assessing postural responses. An important study for clinical investigators.

141. **Raiha I, Luutonen S, Piha J, et al. Prevalence, predisposing factors, and prognostic importance of postural hypotension.** *Arch Intern Med.* **1995;155:930-5.**

Long follow-up of a cohort of older persons showed that orthostatic hypotension was common and could not be ascribed to medications, only to baseline hypertension. Long-term mortality appeared to increase in persons with a significant decrement in diastolic pressure on standing but not in those with systolic decrements; even this association weakened with multivariate analysis, suggesting that the diastolic dip may be a proxy for something else.

142. **Ward C, Kenny RA. Reproducibility of orthostatic hypotension in symptomatic elderly.** *Am J Med.* **1996;100:418-22.**

Shows that in patients with symptomatic orthostatic hypotension, the phenomenon could be reproduced in only 67%. Furthermore, orthostatic hypotension was less prominent when measurements were made in the afternoon rather than the morning, counterintuitively in relation to the sense of postprandial hypotension in elderly persons. Recognition of these caveats is paramount to avoid underestimating orthostatic hypotension in elderly persons.

Pulsus paradoxus

143. **Fowler NO. Physiology of cardiac tamponade and pulsus paradoxus. I: Mechanisms of pulsus paradoxus in cardiac tamponade.** *Mod Concept Cardiovasc Dis.* **1978;47:109-13.**

Although condensed and crowded with small illustrations, this material makes it easier to understand a sign whose comprehension and elicitation pose much difficulty. Further practical advice would be welcome.

144. **Sapira JD, Kirkpatrick MB. On pulsus paradoxus.** *South Med J.* **1983;76:1163-4.**

Brief review of methods to teach the technique of measuring pulsus paradoxus with a sphygmomanometer.

Heart rate and pulse character

145. **D'Cruz IA. Pulsus alternans: a neglected sign of left ventricular failure.** *IM (Internal Medicine for the Specialist).* **1989;10(12):57-9, 62-3, 65.**

Describes elicitation, differential diagnosis, and some physiology, drawing on the author's long study and use of echocardiography.

146. **Hjalmarson A, Gilpin EA, Kjekshus J, et al. Influence of heart rate on mortality after myocardial infarction.** *Am J Cardiol.* **1990;65:547-53.**

Large retrospective study demonstrates heart rate to be a fairly good prognosticator in acute myocardial infarction. A heart rate greater than 90 bpm on admission or at discharge from the hospital was associated with a significant increase in in-hospital and 1-year mortality.

147. **Levine HJ. Optimum heart rate in large failing hearts.** *Am J Cardiol.* **1988;61:633-6.**

Editorial that uses comparative (interspecies) physiology to understand the basis of the bradycardic effect of increased cardiac mass, and to raise the issue of identifying the optimal heart rate in heart failure, something at which we are not yet effective.

148. **Sneed NV, Hollerbach AD. Accuracy of heart rate assessment in atrial fibrillation.** *Heart Lung.* **1992;21(5):427-33.**

Describes how measuring heart rate for 60 seconds is only trivially more accurate than measuring for 15 or 30 seconds, and how apical rate measurement is superior to radial pulse counting. This article contains tons of statistics and fails to account properly for pulse deficit.

149. **Spodick DH. Redefinition of normal sinus heart rate.** *Chest.* **1993;104:939-41.**

It makes sense to move the threshold for bradycardia down from 60 bpm to 50 bpm, and for tachycardia, from 100 bpm to 90 bpm.

Respiratory rate and pattern

150. **Fieselmann JF, Hendryx MS, Helms CM, Wakefield DS. Respiratory rate predicts cardiopulmonary arrest for internal medicine inpatients.** *J Gen Intern Med.* **1993;8:354-60.**

Interesting, thoughtful study. However, much manipulation of numbers is undertaken to support intervening when the respiratory rate exceeds 27 breaths per minute. The predictive value of a positive test is unacceptably low; by the authors' own admission, they would need to evaluate 50 patients to have a chance of benefitting one.

151. **Kesten S, Maleki-Yazdi R, Sanders BR, et al. Respiratory rate during acute asthma.** *Chest.* **1990;97:58-62.**

In spontaneous asthmatic flare-ups there is insufficient correlation with peak expiratory flow rate to serve as a proxy for the test. The authors raise further questions, and the selective amplification of anxiety with dyspnea, in contrast to other symptoms, is not addressed.

152. **Kory RC. Routine measurement of respiratory rate: an expensive tribute to tradition. *JAMA*. 1957;165:448-50.**

Even four decades ago, in only 5% of cases did the physician of record want the information from routine measurements of respiratory rate. When the rate was remeasured by the physician, the measurements of the physician differed so greatly from those done by the nurses that one might feel that the vital sign sheets must have been preprinted "Respiratory rate: 20"!

153. **Mador MJ, Tobin MJ. Apneustic breathing: a characteristic feature of brainstem compression in achondroplasia? *Chest*. 1990;97:877-83.**

Generalizable lesson for recognizing the pattern labeled apneusis, defined as a 3-second pause at the end of inspiration and before expiration begins, a sort of involuntary breath-holding.

154. **Rich MW, Radwany SM. Respiratory dyskinesia: an underrecognized phenomenon. *Chest*. 1994;105:1826-32.**

Two case reports and comprehensive review of this apparently common, albeit seldom recognized, feature of tardive dyskinesia. It is characterized by irregular, rapid breathing, associated with oropharyngeal dyskinesia and respiratory alkalosis. Two other clues are its disappearance during sleep and its usual occurrence in persons with manifest conventional tardive dyskinesia. As with periodic breathing (*see* Liippo, reference 155), this pattern is often misinterpreted.

Periodic breathing (Cheyne-Stokes respiration)

155. **Liippo K, Puolijoki H, Tala E. Periodic breathing imitating hyperventilation syndrome. *Chest*. 1992;102:638-9.**

This single-case study adds capnography to the means whereby one can avoid misinterpreting the hyperpneic phase of Cheyne-Stokes respiration as psychogenic hyperventilation. It is a trap that every experienced clinician has seen. Awareness and vigilance would seem to offer full protection without the need for technology, except in the rarest of circumstances.

156. **Ribeiro JP, Knutzen A, Rocco MB, et al. Periodic breathing during exercise in severe heart failure: reversal with milrinone or cardiac transplantation. *Chest*. 1987;92:555-6.**

Important insights about the mysterious Cheyne-Stokes breathing pattern, including its precipitability with exercise and its reversal with therapy.

157. **Yajima T, Koike A, Sugimoto K, et al. Mechanism of periodic breathing in patients with cardiovascular disease.** *Chest.* **1994;106:142-6.**

A technology-intensive study showing that fluctuation in pulmonary blood flow may underlie the periodic (Cheyne-Stokes) respiratory pattern in heart failure. Surely not the last word on the subject.

The "fifth vital sign": oximetry

158. **Ries AL, Prewitt LM, Johnson JJ. Skin color and ear oximetry.** *Chest.* **1989;96:287-90.**

Pulse oximeters often cannot capture a good signal in patients with a darker complexion when compared with subjects with lighter skin. The authors suggest a lower accuracy of measurement in the former group, but the analysis of data presented does not permit this conclusion.

Skin

General material and textbooks

159. Anonymous. **Skin surface microscopy: anything new under the sun?** [Leading article]. *Lancet.* **1989;1:1239.**

    In American practice, there is a new, higher-intensity light that seems to be favored for use in close inspection. Time will tell whether the light really enhances diagnosis, particularly differential diagnosis of pigmented lesions, or whether it is a gimmick.

160. **Fitzpatrick TB, Eisen AZ, Wolff K, et al., eds.** *Dermatology in General Medicine.* **4th ed. New York: McGraw-Hill, Inc.; 1993.**

    The premier textbook on the skin for the internist. Physical diagnosis plays an absolutely pre-eminent part. Far superior to previous editions by virtue of color illustrations that appear on almost every page and that immediately face the lucid and comprehensive text, rather than being sequestered in harder-to-use and less abundant separate color plates.

161. **Fitzpatrick TB, Polano MK, Suurmond D.** *Color Atlas and Synopsis of Clinical Dermatology: Common and Serious Diseases.* **2nd ed. New York: McGraw-Hill; 1994.**

    Capsular text faces each illustration. The photographs are well reproduced in color, abundant, and sufficiently large. One does not feel, as with many dermatology books, that one is missing the "inside story."

162. **Phillips TJ, Dover JS. Recent advances in dermatology (Medical Progress).** *N Engl J Med.* **1992;326:167-78.**

    The illustrations of HIV-associated lesions of skin and mucous membranes are most useful. Also contains discussion of several other classes of lesions, albeit mostly on their etiology and therapy.

163. **Witkowski JA, Parish LC. The touching question.** *Int J Dermatol.* **1981;20:426.**

Discusses how the importance of feeling skin lesions contrasts with how seldom skin palpation is actually performed. The "old" fear of acquiring spirochetes has been supplanted by fear of retroviruses. Points out that there is no reason one cannot feel successfully through a glove when working around the anus or genitals or when dealing with open skin lesions any place on the body, and no reason a glove is needed if one is *not* dealing with the anus, genitals, or open skin lesions.

Nonmelanocytic skin cancers

164. **Kopf AW, Salopek TG, Slade J, et al. Techniques of cutaneous examination for the detection of skin cancer.** *Cancer.* **1995;75(2 Suppl):684-90.**

Passionately and wisely advocates exposure and inspection of all skin, with the patient wearing no clothing or cosmetics. Describes and illustrates a sequence of examination that ensures seeing all areas, including toe webs, heels, and the lairs of melanoma on the back and legs. Mentions Wood's light, dermoscopy (epi-illumination with oil), standardized photography, and patient education about sunlight as a carcinogen.

165. **Preston DS, Stern RS. Nonmelanoma cancers of the skin (Medical Progress).** *N Engl J Med.* **1992;327:1649-62.**

Although only the second quarter addresses bedside diagnosis, the quality of the numerous color illustrations and their captions makes this a substantive source of help for the internist seeking better discrimination between innocuous lesions and those troublesome ones that require referral.

Pigmented and melanocytic lesions

166. **Boyce JA, Bernhard JD. Routine total skin examination to detect malignant melanoma.** *J Gen Intern Med.* **1987;2:59-61.**

Describes how looking at all of the skin increases yield sufficiently to be worthwhile.

167. **Cassileth BR, Lusk EJ, Guerry D IV, et al. "Catalyst" symptoms in malignant melanoma.** *J Gen Intern Med.* **1987;2:1-4.**

Discusses how certain symptoms cause patients and doctors to take action. Unfortunately, most symptoms occur relatively late, when surgery is no longer likely to result in cure.

168. Fitzpatrick TB, Gilchrest BA. **Dimple sign to differentiate benign from malignant pigmented cutaneous lesions.** *N Engl J Med.* 1977;296:1518.

Unfortunately, only separates dermatofibroma from melanocytic lesions, not nevi from melanomas. May help in deciding whether to do a biopsy.

169. Friedman RJ, Rigel DS. **The clinical features of malignant melanoma.** *Dermatol Clin.* 1985;3:271-83.

A list and discussion of characteristics that help in the decision of who needs biopsy or dermatologic referral.

170. Friedman RJ, Rigel DS, Kopf AW. **Early detection of malignant melanoma: the role of physician examination and self-examination of the skin.** *CA Cancer J Clin.* 1985;35:130-51.

Color atlas and brief text on melanoma and its mimics, including dysplastic nevi. Illustrations of mimics, early melanomas, and dysplastic nevi represent advances over previous fine atlases.

171. Kelly JW, Crutcher WA, Sagebiel RW. **Clinical diagnosis of dysplastic melanocytic nevi: a clinicopathologic correlation.** *J Am Acad Dermatol.* 1986;14:1044-52.

See combined review in reference 172.

172. Rhodes AR. Acquired dysplastic melanocytic nevi and cutaneous melanoma: precursors and prevention. *Ann Intern Med.* 1985;102:546-8.

Both this paper and reference 171 focus on the entity but may not bring the internist to the point of feeling confident in making the diagnosis, even tentatively.

173. Koh HK. **Cutaneous melanoma (Medical Progress).** *N Engl J Med.* 1991;325:171-82.

Excellent color illustrations as well as clear discussion of recent exciting developments in early diagnosis, which is associated with an extremely high cure rate, in stark contrast to the cure rate associated with late-stage disease.

Skin signs of systemic disease and skin involvement in systemic disease

General signs and neoplasia

174. Braverman IM. *Skin Signs of Systemic Disease.* 2nd ed. Philadelphia: WB Saunders; 1981.

Indispensable, although anecdotal, argumentative, and, in places, outdated.

175. **Callen JP. Skin signs of internal malignancy: fact, fancy and fiction.** *Semin Dermatol.* **1984;3:340-57.**

This summary article, full of color pictures, caps the entire issue devoted to the topic. It studies the evidence, explodes false associations (for example, shingles), and validates true ones (for example, acanthosis nigricans).

176. **Callen JP, Jorizzo JL, Greer KE, et al, eds.** *Dermatological Signs of Internal Disease,* **2nd ed. Philadelphia: WB Saunders; 1995.**

Up-to-date, thoughtful chapters on a wide variety of topics. Not so encyclopedic as Braverman's book (reference 174).

177. **Ellis DL, Kafka SP, Chow JC, et al. Melanoma, growth factors, acanthosis nigricans, the sign of Leser-Trélat, and multiple acrochordons: a possible role for alpha-transforming growth factor in cutaneous paraneoplastic syndromes.** *N Engl J Med.* **1987;317:1582-7.**

Employs laboratory investigation by sophisticated methods as one element in an ambitious attempt to define biochemical commonalities in these seemingly diverse settings.

Gastrointestinal and hepatobiliary disorders

178. **Radack K, Park S. Is there a valid association between skin tags and colonic polyps: insights from a quantitative and methodologic analysis of the literature.** *J Gen Intern Med.* **1993;8:413-21.**

Problems with past studies mean that we still do not know the answer. At present, we cannot infer an increased likelihood of polyps based on the presence of skin tags. We believe that more generalizable and rigorous studies may lead to clearer guidelines.

179. **Venencie PY, Cuny M, Samuel D, Bismuth H. The "butterfly" sign in patients with primary biliary cirrhosis [Letter].** *J Am Acad Dermatol.* **1988;19:571-2.**

The "butterfly" sign is an area on the back that the patient cannot reach with his or her finger to scratch. It occurs in the setting of extreme, protracted, generalized pruritus. This island, free of postinflammatory hyperpigmentation, can easily be misconstrued as a local abnormality rather than as the only region that has been spared excoriation.

Vasculitides and hematologic disorders

180. Asherson RA. Subungual splinter hemorrhages: a new sign of the antiphospholipid antibody? [Letter]. *Ann Rheum Dis.* 1990;49:268.

Discusses how florid, otherwise unexplained, "splinters" may be seen in this condition. Does not serve as a good sign of the antiphospholipid antibody syndrome because of very high background prevalence of splinter hemorrhages from trauma and in normal persons.

181. Auletta MJ, Headington JT. Purpura fulminans: a cutaneous manifestation of severe protein C deficiency. *Arch Dermatol.* 1988;124:1387-91.

Clinical description and pathophysiologic exploration.

182. Bickers DR. The dermatologic manifestations of human porphyria. *Ann N Y Acad Sci.* 1987;514:261-7.

Relatively straightforward account, although a little overwhelming for the reader who cannot reel off the variants of porphyria.

183. Carmel R. Hair and fingernail changes in acquired and congenital pernicious anemia. *Arch Intern Med.* 1985;145:484-5.

Brief case reports of striking, uncommon features in two highly atypical patients. The author has published extensively in the field of vitamin B_{12} deficiencies.

184. Grob JJ, Bonerandi JJ. Cutaneous manifestations associated with the presence of the lupus anticoagulant. *J Am Acad Dermatol.* 1986;15:211-9.

Discusses how leg ulcers resembling pyoderma gangrenosum, acral ischemia, including that at fingertips, and livedo reticularis seem to be associated with the antiphospholipid syndrome.

185. Piette WW, Stone MS. A cutaneous sign of IgA-associated, small dermal vessel leukocytoclastic vasculitis in adults (Henoch-Schönlein purpura). *Arch Dermatol.* 1989;125:53-6.

Plaques of palpable purpura with multifocal hemorrhagic and necrotic zones within them, in seven patients assessed by a major authority.

186. Strobach RS, Anderson SK, Doll DC, Ringenberg QS. The value of the physical examination in the diagnosis of anemia: correlation of the physical findings and the hemoglobin concentration. *Arch Intern Med.* 1988;148:831-2.

In addition to the other findings, this straightforward research shows that the palmar creases can become pale well above the widely touted level of 7 g/dL.

187. Weinstein C, Littlejohn GO, Miller MH, et al. **Lupus and non-lupus cutaneous manifestations in systemic lupus erythematosus.** *Aust N Z J Med.* 1987;17:501-6.

Among 84 patients with lupus who were studied closely and who often underwent skin biopsy, both lupus-related and lupus-independent rashes were common. Among malar rashes in this group, seborrheic dermatitis and essential telangiectasia of the malar area were the most common mimics of lupus malar rash.

Infectious diseases and fever

188. Friedman-Kien AE. *Color Atlas of AIDS.* **Philadelphia: WB Saunders; 1989.**

Covers the dermatologic aspects of AIDS, especially Kaposi sarcoma, with remarkable depth and authority. Spotty on other physical signs, such as retinal and oral signs.

189. Schlossberg D. **Fever and rash.** *Infect Dis Clin North Am.* **1996;10:101-10.**

Review of this ever-important topic, with discussion of the petechial, maculopapular, vesiculobullous, erythematous, and urticarial subtypes.

Endocrine diseases

190. Bunker CB, Newton JA, Kilborn J, et al. **Most women with acne have polycystic ovaries.** *Br J Dermatol.* **1989;121:675-80.**

The correlation of acne with polycystic ovaries by ultrasound is intriguing, but the authors acknowledge that many of the patients show an absence of the hormonal syndrome implied in the name. One is left wondering what to do with this report.

191. Feingold KR, Elias PM. **Endocrine-skin interactions: cutaneous manifestations of pituitary disease, thyroid disease, calcium disorders, and diabetes.** *J Am Acad Dermatol.* **1987;17:921-40.**

Long and hard to read through but a helpful reference work.

192. Fiorini A. **A complication of capillary glucose monitoring.** *BMJ.* **1986;293:597-8.**

Case report of striking gangrene of a pulp tip that was excessively used for fingerstick glucose monitoring in a patient with microvasculopathy. The physical finding itself, although familiar, looks out of place—namely, it is expected in a toe instead. Sound suggestions for avoiding this problem.

193. Lowitt MH, Dover JS. Necrobiosis lipoidica (Continuing medical education). *J Am Acad Dermatol.* 1991;25:735-48.

Review of this still ill-understood entity, which is no longer tied as closely to diabetes mellitus as it used to be. Complete with color illustrations of both clinical lesions and histopathologic bases.

194. McKenna TJ. Screening for sinister causes of hirsutism [Editorial]. *N Engl J Med.* 1994;331:1015-6.

Features that warrant the biochemical search for, and imaging studies directed toward, the tiny subset of women with hirsutism who have major endocrinopathies or neoplasms: those in whom it has been present for less than 1 year; those who, at the time of onset, were not 15 to 25 years old (the age group in which most cases of most polycystic ovary syndrome and of idiopathic hirsutism present); and those with virilizing signs such as clitoromegaly, frontal balding, deepening of the voice, or features of associated Cushing's syndrome.

Miscellaneous material

195. Bernhard JD. Auspitz sign is not sensitive or specific for psoriasis. *J Am Acad Dermatol.* 1990;22:1079-81.

Discusses how the removal of a scale causes pinpoint bleeding in fewer than one fifth of patients in whom psoriasis has been established, and occurs in other scaling processes, including the ubiquitous seborrheic keratosis. Another physical sign that no longer earns its keep.

196. Fried M, Kahanovich S, Dagan (Reiss) R. Enoxaparin-induced skin necrosis [Letter]. *Ann Intern Med.* 1996;125:521-2.

The latest in the long list of idiosyncratic vasculitic drug reactions. This reaction occurred due to use of the low-molecular-weight heparins that are increasingly being used.

197. Requena L, Requena C, Sanchez M, et al. Chemical warfare: cutaneous lesions from mustard gas. *J Am Acad Dermatol.* 1988; 19:529-36.

Although we deplore those responsible for such inhumanities, the study of patients gassed in the Iran-Iraq war of the 1980s—using the same agent dreaded in World War I—enhances the physician's ability to help war victims and those receiving therapeutic topical nitrogen mustard.

Nails and clubbing

198. **Armitage KB, Fisher ME. Pitting edema and hypertrophic pulmonary osteoarthropathy [Letter].** *Arch Intern Med.* **1989;149:223, 227.**

Case report and consideration of a rarely recognized association: Hypertrophic pulmonary osteoarthropathy can produce pitting edema.

199. **Beaven DW, Brooks SE.** *Color Atlas of the Nail in Clinical Diagnosis.* **2nd ed. St. Louis: Mosby–Year Book; 1994.**

Succinct text and large, clear photographs focus predominantly on meaningful issues, not minutiae.

200. **Cordasco EM Jr, Beder S, Coltro A, et al. Clinical features of the yellow nail syndrome.** *Cleve Clin J Med.* **1990;57:472-6.**

Insightful discussion about mechanism, linked to individual case studies.

201. **Davis GM, Rubin J, Bower JD. Digital clubbing due to secondary hyperparathyroidism.** *Arch Intern Med.* **1990;150:452-4.**

Discusses still another cause of clubbing.

202. **Hansen-Flaschen J, Nordberg J. Clubbing and hypertrophic osteoarthropathy.** *Clin Chest Med.* **1987;8:287-98.**

Reviews pulmonary and extrapulmonary causes as well as details of diagnostic technique. Thirteen other articles round out this issue of this journal, which is devoted to pulmonary signs and symptoms.

203. **Holzberg M, Walker HK. Terry's nails: revised definition and new correlations.** *Lancet.* **1984;1:896-9.**

Updated criteria and subsequent re-examination of the meaning of the sign.

204. **Kenik JG, Maricq HR, Bole GG. Blind evaluation of the diagnostic specificity of nailfold capillary microscopy in the connective tissue diseases.** *Arthritis Rheum.* **1981;24:885-91.**

Large-scale illustrations and concise text on the technique, which can help in the diagnosis of dermatomyositis, progressive systemic sclerosis, and benign Raynaud's disease.

205. Minkin W, Rabhan NB. Office nail fold capillary microscopy using ophthalmoscope. *J Am Acad Dermatol.* 1982;7:190-3.

Discusses the use of an ophthalmoscope to the same end. Less unwieldy than a microscope but probably also less reliable.

206. **Lampe RM, Kagan A. Detection of clubbing: Schamroth's sign. Closing the window and opening the angle.** *Clin Pediatr.* **1983;22:125.**

Brief extension, from adult medicine to pediatrics, of a new sign for clubbing, first described by a physician on himself.

207. **Muehrcke RC. The finger-nails in chronic hypoalbuminaemia: a new physical sign.** *BMJ.* **1956;1:1327-8, plus figures.**

Wonderfully creative and astute description of the paired white lines that clear with correction of severe hypoalbuminemia but do not grow out. A model of how to conduct clinical research.

208. **Verghese A, Krish G, Howe D, Stonecipher M. The harlequin nail: a marker for smoking cessation.** *Chest.* **1990;97:236-8.**

Describes how nicotine staining present only in the distal part of the nail means the patient gave up cigarettes weeks to months ago, either from loss of ability to manipulate the cigarette or for some other compelling reason.

Head and Face

209. **Banerjee A. How important is scalp soft tissue injury as a predictor of skull fracture?** *J R Soc Med.* **1991;84:502-3.**

Discusses how fractures of the skull that are nondisplaced may not give palpable bony depression. Deep laceration, even in the absence of a palpable osseous displacement, may justify radiographic investigation.

210. **Keipper VL. Snout suffocation syndrome [Letter].** *N Engl J Med.* **1988;319:1097-8.**

Discusses a facies that will be familiar to nursing home physicians. An insightful physician correlated it with intermittent obstruction of the nares and apneic episodes that could not be explicated by pulmonary function tests.

211. **Model D. Smoker's face: an underrated clinical sign?** *Br Med J.* **1985;291:1760-2.**

A discussion of a readily identifiable constellation of changes in skin and facial features that identifies half of chronic smokers with few or no false-positives. The greatest use may be patient motivation rather than clinical diagnosis. Features include gaunt look, leathery skin, excessive skin wrinkling, and both grey and unduly ruddy skin hues.

212. **Van Dooren BT, Van Bruggen AC, Mooij JJ, et al. Noisy intracranial tumours.** *Acta Neurochirurgica.* **1994;131:215-22.**

Intriguing study, using sophisticated microphones attached to the eyelids and computer processing of their signals. Tumor noises were compared with neuroimaging and histologic characteristics, but could not be distinguished from noises associated with intracranial aneurysms or from some noise in some normal persons. Unfortunately, bedside applicability seems remote because the conventional stethoscope has no place in the research.

Sinus examination

213. **Williams JW Jr, Simel DL. Does this patient have sinusitis? Diagnosing acute sinusitis by history and physical examination. (The Rational Clinical Examination.)** *JAMA.* **1993;270:1242-6.**

A very well-balanced review of the value and limitations of the history and examination in the evaluation of acute sinusitis.

214. **Williams JW Jr, Simel DL, Roberts LR, Samsa GP. Clinical evaluation for sinusitis: making the diagnosis by history and physical examination.** *Ann Intern Med.* **1992;117:705-10.**

When present in combination, five history and examination findings predict likely acute or subacute sinusitis: history or examination showing purulent nasal discharge, maxillary toothache, poor response to nasal decongestants, and abnormal transillumination. As an important aside, the clinician's impression of the likelihood of disease fared better than the multiple regression model with the above items.

Eyes

General material and textbooks

215. Handler JA, Ghezzi KT. General ophthalmologic examination. *Emerg Med Clin North Am.* **1995;13:521-38.**

A great deal of useful information, including laudable and well-supported calls to test visual acuity and to use mydriatic (pupillodilating) drops. Geared to the practitioner of emergency medicine but can be used by others. The article contains three errors that should be noted (although they do not vitiate this excellent compendium): misstating the defect in Adie's syndrome, the significance of diopter color on the ophthalmoscope, and omitting viremia from the causes of photophobia.

216. Kanski JJ. *Clinical Ophthalmology: A Systematic Approach.* **3rd ed. Oxford: Butterworth-Heinemann; 1994.**

Practical, comprehensible, and useful, although a little bit cut-and-dried. Nevertheless, invaluable to the non-ophthalmologist.

217. Laganowski HC. The examination of the eye. *Practitioner.* **1988;232:109-10, 112-3.**

A brief review, geared to the non-ophthalmologist, with proper emphasis on the underperformed visual acuity test and an anatomic approach from the surface inward.

218. Spalton DJ, Hitchings RA, Hunter PA, eds. *Atlas of Clinical Ophthalmology.* **2nd ed. St. Louis: Mosby–Year Book; 1994.**

The best illustrations anywhere: abundant, large, and clear. Text is also well written, apt, and comprehensible. Worthwhile for every primary care physician, not just for ophthalmologists.

External eye examination

219. Baum J, Chaturvedi N, Netland PA, Dreyer EB. Assessment of intraocular pressure by palpation. *Am J Ophthalmol.* **1995;119:650-1.**

The method here is studied not for the domain in which the internist would most like to use it—to assess ocular hypotension as a possible correlate of intravascular volume depletion—but rather for marked ocular hypertension in glaucoma; it is only moderately effective for the latter.

220. Earnest DL, Hurst JW. Exophthalmos, stare, increase in intraocular pressure, and systolic propulsion of the eyeballs due to congestive heart failure. *Am J Cardiol.* **1970;26:351-4.**

Discusses how, although the findings can mimic Graves' ophthalmopathy, they abate with diuresis, which does not happen in the case of endocrine eye disease.

221. Feldon SE. Graves' ophthalmopathy: is it really thyroid disease? *Arch Intern Med.* **1990;150:948-50.**

There is a host of unanswered questions, some of which relate to the rarity of the complication, while others relate to its occasional progression despite sustained normalization of thyroid hormone and thyroid-stimulating hormone levels with treatment.

222. Lubs ML, Bauer MS, Formas ME, Djokic B. Lisch nodules in neurofibromatosis type I. *N Engl J Med.* **1991;324:1264-6.**

Discusses how the absence of these nodules beyond a certain age excludes the diagnosis of neurofibromatosis type I with a high degree of certainty, even if not with the perfect level of certainty attained in this study. Lisch nodules are often seen without magnification. If macules are observed in the iris with the unaided eye, a slit lamp examination is required to distinguish these from nevi.

223. Huson S, Jones D, Beck L. Ophthalmic manifestations of neurofibromatosis. *Br J Ophthalmol.* 1987;71:235-8.
Discusses Lisch nodules and other findings, including some in the retina.

224. Maganias NH. A new clinical sign for the diagnosis of allergic conjunctivitis: a brief communication. *Ann Allergy.* **1988;61:273-4.**

Describes how, in allergic conjunctivitis, a half moon (or crescent) of redundant, swollen tissue will bulge out when the lower lid is gently tugged downward with the patient facing upward. Corroboration from other investigators is needed.

225. **Maslin K, Talbot W. The red eye.** *N Z Med J.* **1994;107:512-3.**

Thoughtful, concise, and practical delineation of the major subtypes of conjunctivitis and of the other key classes of red eyes, namely corneal ulcers and lesions, acute anterior uveitis, acute angle closure glaucoma, episcleritis, and scleritis.

226. **Werner SC. Modification of the classification of the eye changes of Graves' disease: recommendations of the ad hoc committee of the American Thyroid Association [Letter].** *J Clin Endocrinol Metab.* **1977;44:203-4.**

A modification of the NOSPECS acronym (N = no findings; O = only signs, no symptoms; S = soft tissue involvement; P = proptosis; E = extraocular muscle involvement; C = corneal involvement; S = sight loss), which renders assessment simpler and clearer.

Pupils

227. **Au Y-K, Henkind P. Pain elicited by consensual pupillary reflex: a diagnostic test for acute iritis.** *Lancet.* **1981;2:1254-5.**

Describes an extremely ingenious test for finding the small subset of patients with "red eyes" who do not have simple conjunctivitis. (Circumlimbal sparing in conjunctivitis has been used but is not perfect.) The examiner has the patient close and cover the red eye and then shines a light into the unaffected eye. In this series, when there was consensual pain in the covered eye, the uvea was inflamed. The authors reported 100% sensitivity and 98% specificity in this series.

228. Chong NVH, Murray PI. Pen torch test in patients with unilateral red eye [Letter]. *Br J Gen Pract.* 1993;43:259.

Discussing the same phenomenon of photosensitivity with an inflamed uvea and ciliary body, the authors describe how discomfort is noted when a penlight ("pen torch" is the British term for this) is shined at the affected eye. They note as an aside that illuminating the opposite eye produces no discomfort, owing to consensual iris contraction. This result is in polar opposition to Au's work, which they do not cite and may not know of.

229. **Chesnut RM, Gautille T, Blunt BA, et al. The localizing value of asymmetry in pupillary size in severe head injury: relation to lesion type and location.** *Neurosurgery.* **1994;34:840-6.**

Describes how fewer than half of acute trauma patients with a 3-mm disparity between pupil sizes had a subdural hematoma ipsilaterally, and how half of patients with a major intracranial hemorrhage had no "blown pupil."

230. **Hamilton Craig I. Emergency differentiation of vasovagal syncope from Stokes-Adams attack.** *Am J Cardiol.* **1984;54:1155.**

Claims that pupillodilation occurs in Stokes-Adams attacks but that pupilloconstriction occurs in vasodepressor (vasovagal) syncope. Requires that one accept that secondary sympathetic stimulation always occurs in Stokes-Adams attacks and never in vasovagal attacks, an unproven assumption. Beta-blockade may prevent development of this sign.

231. **Lam BL, Thompson HS, Corbett JJ. The prevalence of simple anisocoria.** *Am J Ophthalmol.* **1987;104:69-73.**

Elegant study of healthy schoolchildren, adults, and elderly persons shows a 19% point prevalence of perceptible anisocoria. The phenomenon is shown by twice this number at least once among 10 trials spread over 1 week. Accounts for frequently imperceptible light reactions of pupils of elderly persons. Several practical suggestions. Prevents overreaction to the title condition, which is neuro-ophthalmologically innocuous.

232. **Landau WM. Clinical neuromythology I. The Marcus Gunn phenomenon: loose canon of neuro-ophthalmology.** *Neurology.* **1988;38:1141-2.**

A road out of the swamp of the swinging flashlight used in doing the test. The long-winded rejoinder months later in the "Letters" section of the same journal did not augment our understanding.

Retina

233. **Bruno A, Jones WL, Austin JK, et al. Vascular outcome in men with asymptomatic retinal cholesterol emboli: a cohort study.** *Ann Intern Med.* **1995;122:249-53.**

Cohort study with historical controls showing that identification of retinal cholesterol emboli (Hollenhorst plaques) is associated with a tenfold increased incidence of stroke over a mean follow-up of 3.4 years. The study has methodologic problems, particularly with the assessment of controls.

234. **Bull DA, Fante RG, Hunter GC, et al. Correlation of ophthalmic findings with carotid artery stenosis.** *J Cardiovasc Surg.* **1992;33:401-6.**

In this study, amaurosis fugax, but not Hollenhorst plaques or ischemic retinopathy, associated with a high incidence of coexistent stenosis of the ipsilateral carotid.

235. **D'Amico DJ. Diseases of the retina.** *N Engl J Med.* **1994;331:95-106.**

Although the focus is on mechanism and therapy, the abundant high-quality color illustrations and the lucid descriptions of diabetic damage, the complications of AIDS, and age-related macular degeneration make this a helpful article in that most difficult domain, funduscopy.

236. **Duane TD, Osher RH, Green WR. White-centered hemorrhages: their significance.** *Ophthalmology.* **1980;87:66-9.**

Histologic confirmation that these retinal hemorrhages represent extravasated fibrin. They occur in diverse situations, such as AIDS, systemic lupus erythematosus, and severe anemia—not just in endocarditis and leukemia.

237. **Fred HL. Requiem for the ophthalmoscope.** *Hosp Pract* **(Office Edition). 1994;29(2):37-8.**

A horror story: housestaff and attending internists routinely omitting funduscopy, even in evaluating new-onset hemiplegia! Benefit: reassures that one's own institution is not uniquely slovenly. Harm: may make this state of things seem more acceptable. We hope that the Mark Twain model of Premature Reports of Demise applies.

238. **Klein R, Klein BEK, Moss SE, Wang Q. Hypertension and retinopathy, arteriolar narrowing, and arteriovenous nicking in a population.** *Arch Ophthalmol.* **1994;112:92-8.**

The severe methodologic problems of this study, including the enrollment of many persons with hypertension in the control group, vitiate the alleged conclusions.

239. **Levin BE. The clinical significance of spontaneous pulsations of the retinal vein.** *Arch Neurol.* **1978;35:37-40.**

This classic, important, well-designed study shows that the presence of pulsations excludes elevated intracranial pressure. The absence of such pulsations does not allow the opposite inference—that is, that the intracranial pressure is elevated.

240. **Margolis KL, Money BE, Kopietz LA, Rich EC. Physician recognition of ophthalmoscopic signs of open-angle glaucoma: effect of an educational program.** *J Gen Intern Med.* **1989;4:296-9.**

Discusses how a simple educational intervention that includes exposure to clear-cut photographs of optic nerveheads subsequently enhanced subjects' recognition on a standardized test.

241. Phillips CI. **Dilate the pupil and see the fundus.** *Br Med J.* 1984; 288:1779-80.

Discusses the importance of using drops. Concisely and clearly stated, including a comment on the prevention of the (vastly overestimated) complications.

242. Sapira JD. **An internist looks at the fundus oculi.** *Dis Mon.* 1984;30(Nov):1-64.

Splendid description and interpretation. Differential diagnoses of common and uncommon retinal findings.

243. Schwarcz TH, Eton D, Ellenby MI, et al. **Hollenhorst plaques: retinal manifestations and the role of carotid endarterectomy.** *J Vasc Surg.* 1990;11:635-41.

Retrospective series of patients with Hollenhorst plaques. Endarterectomy did not alter future frequency of plaques, amaurosis fugax, transient ischemic attacks, or stroke. The low methodologic power of the study must be recognized, although its results mirror recent evidence from other groups.

244. Traboulsi EI, Krush AJ, Gardner EJ, et al. **Prevalence and importance of pigmented ocular fundus lesions in Gardner's syndrome.** *N Engl J Med.* 1987;316:661-7.

Includes color illustrations. The authors assert that the lesions are sufficiently distinctive to enhance diagnosis.

Ears, Nose, and Throat

245. **Brady PM, Zive MA, Goldberg RJ, et al. A new wrinkle to the earlobe crease.** *Arch Intern Med.* **1987;147:65-6.**

Prospective study using coronary angiography shows identical frequency of coronary atherosclerosis in men with and without creases. Explores sources of differing conclusions from some previous studies.

246. Ishii T, Asuwa N, Masuda S, et al. Earlobe crease and atherosclerosis: an autopsy study. *J Am Geriatr Soc.* 1990;38:871-6.

   This study has some methodologic difficulties. A different populace from the above-mentioned study (Brady, reference 245) and with very different conclusions.

247. **Fisher EW, Pfleiderer AG. Is undergraduate otoscopy teaching adequate?—An audit of clinical teaching.** *J R Soc Med.* **1992;85(1):23-5.**

An extracurricular seminar on otoscopy improved students' confidence and some of their skills in this technique.

248. **Hawke M.** *Clinical Pocket Guide to Ear Disease.* **Philadelphia: Lea & Febiger; 1986.**

Brief text and abundant, excellent color photographs, mostly of diseased external canals and tympanic membranes.

249. **Hawke M, Keene M, Alberti PW.** *Clinical Otoscopy: A Text and Colour Atlas.* **Edinburgh: Churchill Livingstone; 1984.**

Excellent reference source. More detail than the nonotologist usually wants, although selective attention to particular topics is useful.

250. **Kaleida PH, Stool SE. Assessment of otoscopists' accuracy regarding middle-ear effusion: otoscopic validation.** *AJDC.* **1992;146:433-5.**

Describes a formal validation program for *pneumatic* otoscopy that allowed clinicians to develop solid skills in the identification of middle-ear effusions, with a gold standard of immediate myringotomy. Unfortunately, the subjects of this study (examiners) and its objects (ears examined) were too detached from clinical practice conditions.

251. Schmidt PH. Patient interrogation and rhinoscopy. *Acta Otorhino-laryngol Belg.* **1979;33:561-5.**

Discusses the distinguishing features of subtypes of allergic rhinitis. Clearer about interviewing than about examination.

Mouth, Jaws, and Salivary Glands

General material and textbooks

252. **Langlais RP, Miller CS.** *Color Atlas of Common Oral Diseases.* **Philadelphia: Lea & Febiger; 1992.**

Excellent color pictures teach and fortify the physician as well as the dentist in making oral diagnoses. Despite the title, rare conditions are depicted and described along with common ones.

253. **Wood NK, Goaz PW.** *Differential Diagnosis of Oral Lesions.* **4th ed. St. Louis: Mosby–Year Book; 1991.**

Comprehensive discussion. Highly lucid and comprehensible even to the physician whose feelings of inadequacy about intraoral disease encompass ignorance and fear. The first, second, and fourth parts of the book are devoted to clinical diagnosis; the third, which is of less interest to physicians, is devoted to radiographic diagnosis.

Technique of examination

254. **Brentnall E. Spatula test for fracture of mandible.** *Aust Fam Physician.* **1992;21:1007.**

Describes a test in which the patient is asked to bite on a tongue blade and to keep it still as the examiner twists the free end. Allegedly, patients with a fracture cannot complete this test because of pain; no data on sensitivity, specificity, or sources of false-positives are offered.

255. **Eisenberg E, Barasch A. Oral examination: pointers for spotting local and systemic disease.** *Consultant.* **1995;35:1710-21.**

A very brief but useful compendium of techniques, findings, and interpretations.

256. Friedman IH. Say "ah" [Letter]. *JAMA*. 1984;251:2086.

Have the patient sing "Ah!" in falsetto to augment visualization of oral and pharyngeal structures, patient comfort, or both.

Almost as many letters have been published on this topic over the years as on physical signs of handedness. Some useful ones include the following:

257. Greally JM. Alternative to "aaah" [Letter]. *Lancet*. 1988;1:539.

Hold the neck in slight extension, open wide, inspire deeply, and hold the breath *in*!

258. Moore MJ. Say "ah" [Letter]. *JAMA*. 1984;251:2086.

Advocates a loud "Ha!" repeated several times with the tongue drawn as far inward as possible.

259. Savitt JN. "Say ae" [Letter]. *N Engl J Med*. 1976;294:1068-9.

Describes how having the patient say "cat" or "hat" provides a better exposure, if one can ever get patients to use it—a formidable feat even with repetitive personal demonstrations.

Oral cancer

260. Mashberg A, Samit AM. Early detection, diagnosis, and management of oral and oropharyngeal cancer. *CA Cancer J Clin*. 1989;39:67-88.

A map of empirically determined sites of origin differs from widely held conceptions of high-risk areas. Includes classical signs that many physicians already recognize represent advanced disease. Familiarity with subtler signs of earlier cancers should improve outcomes.

261. Mashberg A, Feldman LJ. Clinical criteria for identifying early oral and oropharyngeal carcinoma: erythroplasia revisited. *Am J Surg*. 1988;156:273-5.

A discussion of how red areas are more risky and how invasive cancers are more often granular than in situ cancers.

262. Alvi A. Oral cancer: how to recognize the danger signs. *Postgrad Med*. 1996;99(4):149-56.

Restates the importance of palpation, which may reveal a superficial-looking lesion to be deeply infiltrative. Several illustrations. Despite the title, half of the text concerns therapy.

Other specific oral disorders

263. Correll RW, Wescott WB, Jensen JL. Nonpainful, erythematous, circinate lesions of a protean nature on a fissured tongue. *J Am Dent Assoc*. 1984;109(July):90-1.

Good discussion of benign migratory glossitis (geographic tongue), its association with fissured tongue, the prominent yellow borders that may demarcate it, and its intraoral mimics.

Oral signs of systemic disease and disturbance

264. Beitman RG, Frost SS, Roth JL. Oral manifestations of gastrointestinal disease. *Dig Dis Sci.* **1981;26:741-7.**

Thoughtful coverage of a very broad topic.

265. Benbadis SR, Wolgamuth BR, Goren H, et al. Value of tongue biting in the diagnosis of seizures. *Arch Intern Med.* **1995;155:2346-9.**

A discussion of how a bite laceration on the lateral margin of the tongue is highly specific to generalized tonic-clonic seizure. Because there is so much difficulty with the confounding effect of pseudoseizures, as well as in the seizure-syncope distinction, this sign is most helpful and welcome, despite its low sensitivity.

266. Cunha BA. Crimson crescents—a possible association with the chronic fatigue syndrome [Letter]. *Ann Intern Med.* **1992;116:347.**

Describes how purplish discoloration of the anterior pharyngeal pillars is sometimes seen in the active phase of this condition, without either overt pharyngitis or uvulitis. The crescents fade spontaneously, in tandem with clinical improvement. No biopsy or further characterization is available to date.

267. Drinka PJ, Langer E, Scott L, Morrow F. Laboratory measurements of nutritional status as correlates of atrophic glossitis. *J Gen Intern Med.* **1991;6:137-40.**

Preliminary but intensive study of just two elderly patients, to explore multiple micronutrient status in relation to this sign that in the past has been ascribed to B-vitamin deficiencies.

268. Eisenberg E, Krutchkoff D, Yamase H. Incidental oral hairy leukoplakia in immunocompetent persons: a report of two cases. *Oral Surg Oral Med Oral Pathol.* **1992;74:332-3.**

Satisfactory evidence that even this feared condition occurs, albeit rarely, without immunodeficiency let alone HIV infection.

269. Johnson BE. Halitosis, or the meaning of bad breath. *J Gen Intern Med.* **1992;7:649-56.**

Ill-digested mass of uncritically presented material. Useful for some specific maneuvers for evaluating the process and for some arcane differential diagnoses that are raised, including the psychogenic olfactory reference syndrome.

270. **Lamey P-J, Lewis MAO. Oral medicine in practice: angular cheilitis.** *Br Dent J.* **1989;167:15-8.**

Relation to dentures, candidal infection, and, putatively, to staphylococcal infection. Superior color illustrations, abundant and highly illuminating. An unrealistically intensive routine laboratory work-up is also recommended.

271. **Lockhart PB. Gingival pigmentation as the sole presenting sign of chronic lead poisoning in a mentally retarded adult.** *Oral Surg Oral Med Oral Pathol.* **1981;52:143-9.**

The new twist in this case is the absence of any other recognizable manifestations of plumbism. The implication is that a lead line is worth noting and acting on.

272. **Prema K, Srikantia SG. Clinical grading of lingual lesions in vitamin B-complex deficiency.** *Indian J Med Res.* **1980;72:537-45.**

Includes extremely simple methods, and some attributions based on common sense rather than on scientific proof. This article desperately calls for replication and advance in a setting in which greater technologic correlation is available.

273. **Schneiderman H. Trident tongue of myasthenia gravis.** *Consultant.* **1994;34:367-8.**

Discusses a prototypical "pathognomonic" sign: high specificity, very low sensitivity. A sample of the author's monthly column dealing with topics in physical diagnosis.

274. **Schroeder PL, Filler SJ, Ramirez B, et al. Dental erosion and acid reflux disease.** *Ann Intern Med.* **1995;122:809-15.**

Uses sophisticated methods in support of recognizing yellow dental erosions—not caries—as reason to suspect gastroesophageal reflux disease, for reasons analogous to those for suspecting underlying perimylolysis in persons with bulimia (*see* references 791 and 792).

275. **Talbot T, Jewell L, Schloss E, et al. Cheilitis antedating Crohn's disease: case report and literature update of oral lesions.** *J Clin Gastroenterol.* **1984;6:349-54.**

Describes how the oral mucosa and lips may provide accessible indicators of intestinal lesions. Oral lesions can resemble those in the colon both grossly and microscopically. Occasionally they precede enteric symptoms.

276. Walker JEC. "Serratoglossia" [Letter]. *N Engl J Med.* **1964;271:375.**

Patients with acromegaly and attendant macroglossia can develop a row of indentations on the tip of the tongue. These correspond to pressure, alleviated in the gaps between teeth, that in turn reflects overgrowth of the jaw.

Neck

General material

277. **Hurst JW, Hopkins LC, Smith RB. Noises in the neck.** *N Engl J Med.* **1980;302:862-3.**

Differentiation of carotid bruits from transmitted basal cardiac murmurs, vertebral artery bruits, venous hums, and so on.

278. **Kenna C, Murtagh J. Examination of the neck (2-part article).** *Aust Fam Physician.* **1986;15:1015-20, 1204-12.**

Well-illustrated, concise, and down-to-earth manual for assessment. Despite the title, the second part concerns bedside evaluation of the shoulder, not the neck.

279. **Takahashi K, Groher ME, Michi K-i. Methodology for detecting swallowing sounds.** *Dysphagia.* **1994;9:54-62.**

Exciting, sophisticated, technologically intensive basic science work, geared to clinical utility but not quite "there" yet; see the article by Hamlet and colleagues (reference 22) for additional clinical application.

Specific conditions and signs

280. **Barnett AJ. The "neck sign" in scleroderma.** *Arthritis Rheum.* **1989;32:209-11.**

Selectively ridged and palpably tightened neck skin, brought on by hyperextending the neck, would appear to support the diagnosis strongly, after certain exclusions have been made.

281. **Mizuno A, Yamaguchi K. The plunging ranula.** *Int J Oral Maxillofac Surg.* **1993;22:113-5.**

Shows how this mucus retention phenomenon can present not in the floor of the mouth, where expected, but as a neck mass: it dissects downward from the site of extravasation due to the force of gravity.

282. **Shepherd JJ. Attached to sternomastoid?** *Aust N Z J Surg.* **1979;49:704.**

The examiner has the supine patient actively raise his or her head 1 or 2 inches from the pillow and turn it away from the lump. This will contract both components of the sternomastoid and let the examiner see and feel the relation of the mass to the muscle.

Thyroid examination

283. **Gwinup G, Morton ME. The high lying thyroid: a cause of pseudogoiter.** *J Clin Endocrinol Metab.* **1974;40:37-42.**

Discusses how a normal thyroid lying high in the neck may lead to an unnecessary endocrinologic consultation. If the gland is "a little too prominent" for inspection, but not enlarged enough for palpation, this diagnosis is likely. Imaging can help settle the few instances of this phenomenon that are not clear at the bedside.

284. **Slater S. Palpation of the thyroid gland.** *South Med J.* **1993;86:1001-3.**

Shows that the isthmus is one key to successful palpation, and that the use of anatomic landmarks and inference from the position of the carotid pulse are others.

285. **Wallace C, Siminoski K. The Pemberton sign.** *Ann Intern Med.* **1996;125:568-9.**

A discussion of how large retrosternal goiters can compromise the thoracic inlet. Less severe degrees are revealed by having the patient raise both arms so as to touch the sides of the head, waiting a minute or so, and then observing features of facial congestion and cyanosis as cephalic venous outflow (and sometimes tracheal airflow) is compromised.

Lymph Nodes

286. **Hartveit F, Skarstein A, Varhaug JE. Palpation of the axillary nodes in breast cancer: what does the surgeon feel?** *Breast Cancer Res Treat.* **1988;11:71-5.**

An interesting pathology-based study suggests mechanisms for the well-known problems caused by insensitivity (and nonspecificity) in clinical staging of breast cancer via axillary palpation.

287. **Linet OI, Metzler C. Practical ENT: incidence of palpable cervical nodes in adults.** *Postgrad Med.* **1977;62:210-1, 213.**

Palpable lymph nodes of no lasting significance were detectable in a large percentage of young adults without chronic disease, many of whom had acute upper respiratory tract infections.

288. **Rao PS. Springing test for differentiating a cervical rib tip from a supraclavicular lymph node.** *Jpn J Surg.* **1988;18:606-7.**

A simple method is illustrated: pressing the back of the neck to discover whether the "node" pops; if it does, it has to be attached to where one has pressed—that is, it must be a cervical rib. In this country, however, one might ask, "Why not settle the question with a radiograph?"

289. **Shetty MR. Virchow's node revisited [Letter].** *Arch Otolaryngol Head Neck Surg.* **1988;114:578.**

Makes the single point that any abdominal, pelvic, or intrascrotal cancer, as well as lung cancer, can present with a supraclavicular metastasis as its first clinical manifestation.

Breasts

General material

290. Byrd BF. Close-up: standard breast examination. *CA Cancer J Clin.* **1974;24:290-3.**

Well-illustrated approach.

291. Davis JM. Friction-free BSE. *Penn Med.* **1987;90(1):30, 32.**

Important reminders about physician examination and self-examination, including the value of warm hands and lubricant hand lotion.

292. Fletcher SW, Fletcher RH. The breast is close to the heart [Editorial]. *Ann Intern Med.* **1992;117:969-71.**

Describes internists' tendency to focus on intrathoracic structures of perceived high glamour or utility—the heart and the lungs—at the expense of breast examination. Potently makes a case for why evidence-based medicine dictates that breast examination needs to be a focus for every primary care physician.

293. Mann LC. Physical examination of the augmented breast: description of a displacement technique. *Obstet Gynecol.* **1995;85:290-2.**

Alleges that one can successfully displace the implant with one hand while palpating native breast tissue with the other. Perhaps the best advice is to keep the patient's ipsilateral arm down at her side while palpating supine (rather than overhead as with native breasts), since this tends to keep the implant mobile. The catalogue of diagnostic difficulties, both clinical and mammographic, makes one shake one's head that one million breast implantations have been performed in the United States to date.

294. McKenna RJ Sr, Greene P, Winchester DP, et al. Breast self-examination and breast physical examination. *Cancer.* **1992;69(7 Suppl):2003-4.**

A committee report on present status and prospects for improvement, including simplifying the breast self-examination technique and developing properly illustrated teaching and reinforcement materials such as video-tapes.

295. **Pilgrim C, Lannon C, Harris RP, et al. Improving clinical breast examination training in a medical school: a randomized controlled trial.** *J Gen Intern Med.* **1993;8:685-8.**

Proof of what most clinicians deeply believe almost as a matter of faith: that a practicum, with both silicone breast models and live patients, produces more capable and perhaps more effective breast examinations by medical students than does lecture alone.

296. **Urbani CE, Betti R. Aberrant mammary tissue and nephrourinary malignancy: a man with unilateral polythelia and ipsilateral renal adenocarcinoma associated with polycystic kidney disease.** *Cancer Genet Cytogenet.* **1996;87:88-9.**

Review of the predictive value, noted previously by several other authors, of supernumerary nipples for renal anomalies and renal cell carcinoma. A surface sign of internal disease that merits recognition.

History

297. **Fariselli G, Lepera P, Viganotti G, et al. Localized mastalgia as presenting symptom in breast cancer.** *Eur J Surg Oncol.* **1988;14:213-5.**

Among women with *localized* breast pain but no physical findings, there was a 2.5% prevalence of breast cancer detected by mammography at the site of the pain. In a cohort of women with established breast cancer, a considerable subset had pain at the site before a lump was detected. Although not yet replicated to our knowledge, this is a most provocative study.

Breast cancer, its mimics, and fibrocystic conditions

298. **Baines CJ, Miller AB, Bassett AA. Physical examination: its role as a single screening modality in the Canadian National Breast Screening Study.** *Cancer.* **1989;63:1816-22.**

Focuses on the utility of breast examination by highly trained nurses as compared with that by physicians. Along the way, several other points are discussed, including sensitivity and specificity in relation to histologically proven breast cancer in a cohort that did not receive mammography.

299. **Gump FE, McDermott J. Fibrous disease of the breast in juvenile diabetes.** *N Y State J Med.* **1990;90:356-7.**

This disease produces hard areas that may be subjected to biopsy unnecessarily, according to these authors, who have found characteristic mammographic findings and a context in which the entity is expected.

300. **Hall FM, Connolly JL, Love SM. Lipomatous pseudomass of the breast: diagnosis suggested by discordant palpatory and mammographic findings.** *Radiology.* **1987;5:463-4.**

Discusses the exception to the rule that a negative mammogram does *not* mean a palpable mass is not cancer (*see* reference 303). When the mammogram shows virtually complete replacement of breast tissue by fat, including in the area of palpable pseudomass, the exception may be justifiable.

301. **Heller W, Belmont L. Macromastia in an elderly woman [Letter].** *J Am Geriatr Soc.* **1991;39:107.**

Dependent edema due to congestive heart failure was responsible for the macromastia, with habitual recumbency on one side amplifying the effect. The finding resolved with conservative measures.

302. McElligott G, Harrington MG. Heart failure and breast enlargement suggesting cancer. *Br Med J.* 1986;292:446.

Describes striking abnormality representing local dependent edema. The patient is usually a woman with heart failure who has lain consistently on the affected side.

303. **Langlands AO, Tiver KW. Significance of a negative mammogram in patients with a palpable breast tumour.** *Med J Aust.* **1982;1:30-1.**

Shows the extreme danger of dismissing a breast lump simply because it fails to produce a radiographic density.

304. Hall FM. Screening mammography: potential problems on the horizon. *N Engl J Med.* 1986;314:53-5.

Cites the frequency with which mammography produces false-negative results—that is, the all-important case of false reassurance.

305. **McGinnis LS. The importance of clinical breast examination.** *Cancer.* **1989;64(Suppl 12):2657-60.**

Discusses finger pads; who should perform the examination; technique; and relation to other modes.

306. **Minasian H. The "nodding" sign.** *Ann R Coll Surg Engl.* **1995;77(2):130.**

Very highly specialized. Helps the surgeon choose where to incise: palpation directly over the tip of the needle-localization wire that has been placed mammographically produces maximal "nodding" movement of the free end of the wire emerging from the skin elsewhere.

Gynecomastia

307. **Braunstein GD. Gynecomastia.** *N Engl J Med.* **1993;328:490-5.**

Updates mechanisms and causes, including the many drugs that can produce the finding.

308. **Cavanaugh J, Niewoehner CB, Nuttall FQ. Gynecomastia and cirrhosis of the liver.** *Arch Intern Med.* **1990;150:563-5.**

The mechanisms are not as simple as they might appear.

309. **Wilson JD. Gynecomastia: a continuing diagnostic dilemma.** *N Engl J Med.* **1991;324:334-5.**

Further insight, including an assertion that the cause is more commonly recognized by bedside assessment than by hormonal assays.

Respiratory System

History

310. Schmitt BP, Kushner MS, Wiener SL. The diagnostic usefulness of the history of the patient with dyspnea. *J Gen Intern Med.* 1986;1:386-93.

In an extremely carefully defined situation, faculty members' assignments of causes, based on history alone, were vindicated three times out of four.

Physical examination

Basic science

311. Murphy RL Jr, Holford SK, Knowler WC. Visual lung-sound characterization by time-expanded wave-form analysis. *N Engl J Med.* 1977; 296:968-71.

Brilliant original research that illuminates common bedside findings.

312. Shannon DC. "You see but you do not observe" [Editorial]. *Chest.* 1993;104:1320-1.

Discussion of standardizing methods for lung sound analysis by instrumentation. Not directly helpful for bedside use, although essential to those who wish to further the work of Murphy (*see* reference 311) and to provide further visual insight about auscultatory phenomena.

General material

313. Mulrow CD, Dolmatch BL, Delong ER, et al. Observer variability in the pulmonary examination. *J Gen Intern Med.* 1986;1:364-7.

Particularly well-designed study documents appalling intraobserver and interobserver disagreement about findings. Ends on a hopeful note about the possibility of improvement.

314. **Sharma OP. Symptoms and signs in pulmonary medicine: old observations and new interpretations.** *Dis Mon.* **1995;41:577-638.**

Lengthy but useful. A little excess focus on diseases rather than on individual signs and symptoms, but the abundance of discussion and illustration of extrapulmonary signs in multisystem disorders more than compensates.

315. **Spiteri MA, Cook DG, Clarke SW. Reliability of eliciting physical signs in examination of the chest.** *Lancet.* **1988;i:873-5.**

Methodologically suboptimal study. Suggests alarmingly low interobserver agreement for multiple chest findings, particularly for signs that are either seldom used or rarely present.

Domains other than conventional lung sounds

316. **Baumann MH, Sahn SA. Hammann's sign revisited: pneumothorax or pneumomediastinum?** *Chest.* **1992;102:1281-2.**

Discusses how Hamman's sign may be present in pneumothorax (especially left-sided) as well as in pneumomediastinum. The interaction between the beating heart and trapped air in the pleura seems to generate the sound.

317. **Guarino JR, Guarino JC. Auscultatory percussion: a simple method to detect pleural effusion.** *J Gen Intern Med.* **1994;9:71-4.**

Impressive results of a technique with questionable validity (*see* reference 25 for the arguments). The authors show a sensitivity of 95% and a specificity of 100% of their technique in the detection of pleural effusions. Based on previous experiences with related techniques, these results should be reproduced before being incorporated into routine clinical practice.

318. **Jones FL Jr. Poor breath sounds with good voice sounds: a sign of bronchial stenosis.** *Chest.* **1988;93:312-3.**

Well written, but not yet replicated in other laboratories. May constitute a new reason not to discard intentional transpulmonary auscultation of phonation.

319. **Nelson RS, Rickman LS, Mathews WC, et al. Rapid clinical diagnosis of pulmonary abnormalities in HIV-seropositive patients by auscultatory percussion.** *Chest.* **1994;105:402-7.**

Only other study to echo Guarino's success with auscultatory percussion (*see* reference 317). This technique fared better than auscultation or percussion alone in the detection of radiologic abnormalities. The study group was unique in its huge prevalence of abnormal chest films (55.6%), but this potential source of bias does not render the method inapplicable.

320. Roberts HJ. More on percussion as a way of life [Letter]. *Lancet.* 1995;346:574-5.

Short reflection following notice that the Aye-Aye, a threatened primate in Madagascar, employs percussion in its quest for food. Notes the value of the laying-on of hands, and the interface with technology, as well as the mistreatment of Auenbrugger (*see* reference 21).

321. Sapira JD. About egophony. *Chest.* **1995;108:865-7.**

A sophisticated and informed discussion of both the physics and the perceptual issues, as well as the barriers to using this potentially very helpful modality for evaluating intrathoracic structure.

Lung sounds: general

322. Earis J. Lung sounds. *Thorax.* **1992;47:671-2.**

Brief editorial on the potential mecahnisms of lung sounds.

323. Forgacs P. The functional basis of pulmonary sounds. *Chest.* **1978;73:399-405.**

This excellent summary of pathophysiologic correlations among other things undoes the myth of air bubbling through alveolar fluid as the cause of crackles in pulmonary edema and explicates other pathophysiologic acoustic phenomena.

324. Gilbert VE. True love and auscultations of the lungs [Letter]. *J Tenn Med Assoc.* 1995;88(8):327.

Vignette centered on value of crackles revealed in lateral decubitus position. Moving human reflection as well.

325. Kraman SS. Lung sounds for the clinician. *Arch Intern Med.* **1986; 146:1411-2.**

Tightly written review geared exclusively to clinically useful distinctions.

326. Loudon R, Murphy RL Jr. Lung sounds. *Am Rev Respir Dis.* **1984; 130:663-73.**

In-depth review, oriented toward basic science. New insights about auscultation over the trachea and about measuring and interpreting forced expiratory time.

327. Murphy RL Jr. *A Simplified Introduction to Lung Sounds* **(Audiotape and booklet). Jamaica Plain, Massachusetts: Raymond L. H. Murphy, Jr.; 1977.**

User-friendly booklet and cassette tape. Remains applicable despite the long interval since publication.

328. **Baughman RP, Shipley RT, Loudon RG, Lower EE. Crackles in interstitial lung disease: comparison of sarcoidosis and fibrosing alveolitis. *Chest.* 1991;100:96-101.**

Attempt to identify anatomic features that, with the use of high-resolution computed tomography, would explain the conspicuous paucity of crackles in sarcoidosis when compared with cryptogenic fibrosing alveolitis of similar severity. In our opinion, the answer remains elusive.

329. **Earis JE, Marsh K, Pearson MG, Ogilvie CM. The inspiratory "squawk" in extrinsic allergic alveolitis and other pulmonary fibroses. *Thorax.* 1982;37:923-6.**

Concerns a short, isolated inspiratory sound, typically best heard in the anterior upper chest, which in some cases of diffuse pulmonary fibrosis is heard. It usually coexists with conventional inspiratory crackles. Its separate significance, if any, is unknown.

330. **Nath AR, Capel LH. Inspiratory crackles: early and late. *Thorax.* 1974;29:223-7.**

Crackles confined to the first half of inspiration were found to be associated with severe airways obstruction, whereas those occurring in the second half of inspiration, with or without antecedents in the first half, had no such association. An intriguing and potentially powerful finding. Still awaits corroboration by others more than 2 decades after publication.

331. Nath AR, Capel LH. Inspiratory crackles and mechanical events of breathing. *Thorax.* 1974;29:695-8.
Additional insights, somewhat more general and theoretical, although grounded in empirical data, from the same laboratory.

332. **Piirila P, Sovijarvi ARA, Kaisla T, et al. Crackles in patients with fibrosing alveolitis, bronchiectasis, COPD, and heart failure. *Chest.* 1991; 99:1076-83.**

See combined review in reference 333.

333. **Piirila P. Changes in crackle characteristics during the clinical course of pneumonia. *Chest.* 1992;102:176-83.**

This article and another by Piirila and colleagues (reference 332) show that pneumophonography may identify distinctive features of crackles in lung disease. In one study by Piirila and colleagues (reference 332), crackles were different in the four groups studied, each with particular waveform patterns. In this article (reference 333), crackles were noted to become less intense and to have a later onset in inspiration as pneumonias resolved. Unfortunately, a comparison with stethoscopic auscultation was not made; this could have added clinical applicability to these data. Because pneumophonography is not readily available in most institutions, it is unlikely that the results of these interesting studies will yet have an impact on clinical practice.

334. **Walshaw MJ, Nisar M, Pearson MG, et al. Expiratory lung crackles in patients with fibrosing alveolitis.** *Chest.* **1990;97:407-9.**

Expiratory crackles may be heard in fibrosing alveolitis. They are intermittent (present in only three-fourths of cycles in a group of 13 patients with mild-to-moderate disease) and usually audible in mid-to-late expiration. An inverse correlation between the number of cycles in which expiratory crackles are heard and gas transfer ($r = 0.61$) is shown in this small study.

Obstructive airways disease

335. **Badgett RG, Tanaka DJ, Hunt DK, et al. Can moderate chronic obstructive pulmonary disease be diagnosed by historical and physical findings alone?** *Am J Med.* **1993;94:188-96.**

Among 87 patients, 14 had moderate COPD by spirometric determination. A model containing historical information (previous diagnosis of COPD; a smoking history of 70 pack-years or more) and the finding of decreased breath sounds on examination detected this condition with a sensitivity and specificity of 67% and 98%, respectively. This study is less applicable than that of Holleman (reference 336) because of its more restricted target population. It is interesting to see the interchange of predicting ability between decreased breath sounds and wheezing in the two studies; a possible explanation is the greater severity of disease in this series. A unique strength of this study should be emphasized: 47% of the subjects were women, sharply differing from most other studies in the field.

336. **Holleman DR, Simel DL, Goldberg JS. Diagnosis of obstructive airways disease from the clinical examination.** *J Gen Intern Med.* **1993; 8:63-8.**

In a cohort seen at a Veterans Administration preoperative clinic, a composite model that included smoking history, self-reported wheezing, and auscultated wheezing predicted obstructive airways disease by spirometry with reasonable accuracy (area under the ROC curve, 0.78). Addition of forced expiratory time added little to this value (0.81). A nomogram with these variables was developed and can be used at the bedside to calculate the probabilities of airway obstruction. The careful design and clear writing make this a very worthwhile article.

337. Kern DG, Patel SR. Auscultated forced expiratory time as a clinical and epidemiologic test of airway obstruction. *Chest.* 1991;100:636-9.

See combined review in reference 338.

338. Schapira RM, Schapira MM, Funahashi A, et al. The value of the forced expiratory time in the physical diagnosis of obstructive airways disease. *JAMA.* 1993;270:731-6.

This study and that by Kern and Patel (reference 337) had slightly different populations and definitions for obstructive airways disease. The specificity of this test is limited at any cut-off value; it therefore seems reasonable that one restricts its use only to rule out COPD in patients with a low pre-test probability (by using a lower cut-off point, e.g., 3 seconds), or to confirm it in a patient with high likelihood of disease (by using a high cut-off level, e.g., 12 seconds). The duration of the forced expiratory time does not correlate well with the severity of spirometric airways obstruction ($r = 0.36$ in this series).

339. Kern DG, Patel SR. The diagnostic value of the forced expiratory time [Letter]. *JAMA.* 1994;271:25.

Comments on differences in efficacy between the two studies reviewed jointly above (references 337 and 338), and concludes that the test should not be used at all.

340. Schapira RM, Schapira MM, Funahashi A, et al. The diagnostic value of the forced expiratory time [Letter in reply]. *JAMA.* 1994;271:26.

Explores the cited disparities and advocates a stopwatch rather than a wristwatch to enhance accuracy.

341. Cross HD. Diagnosing obstructive airways disease from the clinical examination [Letter]. *JAMA.* 1995;274:213.

Claims that peak flow measurements are far more useful than bedside examination.

342. Holleman DR Jr. Diagnosing obstructive airways disease from the clinical examination [Letter in reply]. *JAMA.* 1995;274:213-4.

Cites data refuting the assertion.

343. King DK, Thompson BT, Johnson DC. Wheezing on maximal forced exhalation in the diagnosis of atypical asthma: lack of sensitivity and specificity. *Ann Intern Med.* 1989;110:451-5.

A central and unproven assumption is that methacholine sensitivity equals bronchoreactivity. If exceptions exist (such as, perhaps, exercise-induced asthma), the conclusions here will be inapplicable—in which case this sign is not yet ready for the dustbin.

344. Li JTC, O'Connell EJ. Clinical evaluation of asthma. *Ann Allergy Asthma Immunol.* 1996;76:1-14.

Thoughtful, thorough review of both history and physical examination in relation to presence and severity of asthma. Gives these modalities more credit than do some other authors referenced in this bibliography. Concludes that bedside skills ought to be retained and refined, but that spirometry is needed for accurate diagnosis.

345. **Mannino DM, Etzel RA, Flanders WD. Do the medical history and physical examination predict low lung function?** *Arch Intern Med.* **1993;153:1892-7.**

Immense study evaluating 4461 veterans with a questionnaire, physical examination, and spirometry. The authors conclude that the history and examination are inadequate to detect "low lung function," defined as an $FEV_1 < 81.2\%$ of the predicted value. Although the conclusions seem discordant with those of Holleman (*see* reference 336) and of Badgett (*see* reference 335), the statistical analyses and definitions of abnormalities differ, and the negative predictive values of the information were not emphasized. In truth, the data are more neutral, but the interpretations vary more. The reader must draw personal conclusions by reading the data closely.

346. **Mulrow CD, Lucey CR, Farnett LE. Discriminating causes of dyspnea through clinical examination.** *J Gen Intern Med.* **1993;8:383-92.**

Analytical review of a topic in which methodology is a constant problem. With this caveat in mind, the quality and insight of the comments are excellent.

Heart

General material

347. Abrams J. *Essentials of Cardiac Physical Diagnosis.* **Philadelphia: Lea & Febiger; 1987.**

Splendid textbook; covers not only essentials but a great many fine points.

348. Hurst JW. The examination of the heart: the importance of initial screening. *Dis Mon.* **1990;36:249-313.**

A recognized Old Master discusses several issues. The recommended assessment would be considered too lengthy for screening by many readers. Nevertheless, extremely valuable.

349. Nassar ME. The stethoscopeless cardiologist. *J R Soc Med.* **1988;81:501-2.**

A report of an encounter that would be dismissed as hyperbolic if presented in fiction.

350. Perloff JK. The physiologic mechanisms of cardiac and vascular physical signs. *J Am Coll Cardiol.* **1983;1:184-98.**

Excellent use of original descriptions. So compressed that it best serves advanced readers.

History

351. Alpert JS. The patient with angina: the importance of careful listening. *J Am Coll Cardiol.* **1988;11:27.**

Even with coronary angiogram in hand, the history further distinguishes risk.

352. **Klein HO, Nuriel H, Levi A, et al. Pronus angina (angina pectoris induced by stooping or crouching): a proposed mechanism.** *Chest.* **1993; 104:65-70.**

Provides evidence to substantiate the idea that increased afterload is the primary mechanism responsible for the unusual variant of angina upon stooping.

353. **Wellens HJ, Brugada P. Antiarrhythmic therapy: the value of the history of the patient.** *Eur Heart J.* **1987;8:71-5.**

Somewhat disjointed, but useful in describing both the variety of symptoms and the rarity with which some are recognized as arrhythmic in origin.

Nonauscultatory components

354. **Abrams J. Precordial motion in health and disease.** *Modern Concepts of Cardiovascular Disease.* **1980;49:55-60.**

Elegant mixture of technique, physiology, and interpretation.

355. **Eilen SD, Crawford MH, O'Rourke RA. Accuracy of precordial palpation for detecting increased left ventricular volume.** *Ann Intern Med.* **1983;99:628-30.**

Discusses how enlargement of the apical impulse means more than displacement. Application requires excluding myocardial hypertrophy, something beyond the power of physical examination. Sober conclusions after a fine study of a difficult topic.

356. **Heckerling PS, Wiener SL, Moses VK, et al. Accuracy of precordial percussion in detecting cardiomegaly.** *Am J Med.* **1991;91:328-34.**

In a closely defined group, this formerly discredited maneuver showed powerful predictive value, particularly when used with discrete and well-chosen points on a receiver operating characteristic curve.

357. **Heckerling PS, Wiener SL, Wolfkiel CJ, et al. Accuracy and reproducibility of precordial percussion and palpation for detecting increased left ventricular end-diastolic volume and mass.** *JAMA.* **1993;270:1943-8.**

In a group with a high prevalence of heart disease, percussion of the left cardiac border had a high sensitivity and negative predictive value to detect left ventricular enlargement compared with a gold standard of ultrafast cardiac computed tomography. Specificity was quite low, but the former operating characteristics may suffice to justify the use of percussion and palpation to exclude cardiomegaly.

358. Spodick DH. Accuracy of precordial percussion and palpation [Letter]. *JAMA.* 1994;271:1318-9. See combined review in reference 359.

359. Heckerling PS, Wiener SL, Kushner MS. Accuracy of precordial percussion and palpation [Letter]. *JAMA.* 1994;271:1319.

This accompanying correspondence to the letter of Spodick (reference 358) addresses our main concern: degree of interobserver variability, especially for precordial palpation.

360. Karnegis JN, Kadri N. Accuracy of percussion of the left cardiac border. *Int J Cardiol.* 1992; 37:361-4.

Discusses how estimation of the left cardiac border by percussion is correct within 1 cm in 74% of examinations, using an anteroposterior supine chest film as the gold standard, with reasonable inter-rater agreement. Although this study uses less sophisticated methods, it nonetheless corroborates some of Heckerling's findings (*see* reference 356).

361. Heinz GJ III, Zavala DC. Slipping rib syndrome: diagnosis using the "hooking maneuver." *JAMA.* 1977;237:794-5.

Describes a surprisingly little-used method by which one precisely reproduces chest or abdominal pain caused by slipping ribs, by pulling the lower ribs anteriorly.

362. O'Neill TW, Barry M, Smith M, Graham IM. Diagnostic value of the apex beat. *Lancet.* 1989;i:410-1.

Discusses how palpation of the apex beat beyond the left mid-clavicular line has limited sensitivity (59%) but better specificity (76%) to detect radiographic cardiomegaly. A prominent effect of body habitus on apex palpability must not be underestimated. Some readers find the evidence more persuasive than do other readers.

363. Parrino TA. Hands on the heart: palpation of the cardiovascular system. *Hosp Pract.* 1989;24(4A):103-15.

Scholarly and engaging presentation of information on palpation of arteries and the heart, employing the focus of a general internist rather than of a cardiologist.

Auscultation

General

364. Craige E. Should auscultation be rehabilitated? [Editorial]. *N Engl J Med.* 1988;318:1611-3.

A beautiful essay that provides several major components of an affirmative answer to the title question. Lucid consideration of the technology-examination interface in general.

365. **Harvey WP, Canfield DC.** *Clinical Auscultation of the Cardiovascular System: High Fidelity Recordings of More Than 450 Actual Patients with Companion Texts.* **Newton, New Jersey: Laennec Publishing; 1989.**

Extends the impact of this acknowledged world authority by including audible examples to accompany insightful words. One must listen to the audio examples on a good system, not in the car.

366. Harvey WP. Cardiac pearls: masters in medicine. *Dis Mon.* 1994;40:43-113.

Legendary Dr. Harvey leisurely presents insights from his almost 50 years of cardiology practice. With no references and abundant anecdotes, the article reads like a transcript from bedside rounds with the maestro. Far more useful is the mixed-media material cited in reference 365.

367. **Reddy PS, Haidet K, Meno F. Relation of intensity of cardiac sounds to age.** *Am J Cardiol.* **1985;55:1383-8.**

Phonocardiographic evidence that S1 and S3, but not S4, decrease in intensity with aging.

368. **Shaver JA. Cardiac auscultation: a cost-effective diagnostic skill.** *Curr Probl Cardiol.* **1995;20:441-530.**

Once one finishes choking over the premise that it needs to be proved that cardiac auscultation is cost effective, one can enjoy the potent introductory material demonstrating this premise, and the delightful drawings by Ernest Craige, the first of which is captioned, "Often before an adequate history and physical examination have been performed, the patient is placed on the conveyor belt of diagnostic tests and procedures." The review of auscultation reflects the authority and lucidity of the esteemed Dr. Shaver.

Auscultatory manipulations and maneuvers

369. **Lembo NJ, Dell'Italia LJ, Crawford MH, O'Rourke RA. Diagnosis of left-sided regurgitant murmurs by transient arterial occlusion: a new maneuver using blood pressure cuffs.** *Ann Intern Med.* **1986;105:368-70.**

A brilliantly executed study of a simple manipulation that avoids the hazards, false-positive results, and requirements for spry or cooperative patients that plague several other alternatives. Specifically, blood pressure cuffs are placed on both arms, inflated to 100 mm Hg, and the effect on the murmur is observed. Be sure to deflate promptly afterward!

370. **Maisel AS, Atwood JE, Goldberger AL. Hepatojugular reflux: useful in the bedside diagnosis of tricuspid regurgitation.** *Ann Intern Med.* **1984; 101:781-2.**

Discusses the combined use of this maneuver—better dubbed "the abdominal pressure test" (*see* reference 453)—and of the Carvallo sign, to augment a murmur; provides excellent sensitivity and specificity.

371. Gooch AS, Cha SD, Maranhao V. The use of the hepatic pressure maneuver to identify the murmur of tricuspid regurgitation. *Clin Cardiol.* 1983;6:277-80.

Additional investigation of closely related issues.

372. **Nishimura RA, Tajik AJ. The Valsalva maneuver and response revisited.** *Mayo Clin Proc.* **1986;61:211-7.**

Superb review of a maneuver that often receives suboptimal attention in standard textbooks. The authors describe in detail its use in the evaluation of autonomic dysfunction, cardiac murmurs, and a few other, unusual situations.

373. **Perry GY, Pitlik S, Greenwald M, Rosenfeld JB. Cardiac auscultation of "bony" chests.** *Isr J Med Sci.* **1984;20:260-1.**

Interposition of 150-mL plastic infusion bag, 80% full of saline solution, achieves an acoustic seal so that bell or diaphragm can be used effectively.

374. **Rothman A, Goldberger AL. Aids to cardiac auscultation.** *Ann Intern Med.* **1983;99:346-53.**

Does not catalogue such maneuvers. For example, passive straight-leg raising is not mentioned. Rather, it critiques methods and studies defining specificity of responses to any maneuver. The work of Lembo (*see* reference 394) furthers this effort, but much additional investigation is needed to provide generalizable conclusions.

375. **Tan L-B, McGladdery SL, Meyer T. Simple bedside aid to cardiac auscultation [Letter].** *Lancet.* **1990;335:1031.**

Description of the use of a plastic 20-mL syringe to facilitate the bedside performance of the Valsalva and Muller maneuvers.

376. **Wang K, Hodges M. The premature ventricular complex as a diagnostic aid.** *Ann Intern Med.* **1992;117:766-70.**

Concise, useful article on some of the diagnostic uses of premature ventricular complexes. In the case of physical diagnosis, their value includes the differential diagnosis of systolic murmurs, the unmasking of pulsus alternans, and the distinction between S3 and S4.

First and second heart sounds

377. **Adolph RJ, Fowler NO. Second heart sound: a screening test for heart disease.** *Modern Concepts of Cardiovascular Disease.* **1970;39:91-6.**

An extremely easy to understand and well-written article that remains as useful now as when first published over a quarter of a century ago.

Third and fourth heart sounds

378. Benchimol A, Desser KB. The fourth heart sound in patients without demonstrable heart disease. *Am Heart J.* 1977;93:298-301.

A fourth sound was heard in 60 of 100 consecutive patients with normal invasive studies of both right-heart and left-heart structure and function. Reviews the controversy and consequences of upsetting an entrenched interpretative error. Loud S4s may have more significance.

379. Folland ED, Kriegel BJ, Henderson WG, et al. Implications of third heart sounds in patients with valvular heart disease. *N Engl J Med.* 1992;327:458-62.

Large study which, although not designed specifically for the evaluation of S3 (as evidenced by the limitations in data retrieval), improves our insights on S3 in pathologic states. An S3 was associated with indices of left ventricular dysfunction in patients with aortic stenosis and mixed aortic valve disease, but not in patients with isolated mitral or aortic regurgitation. In this latter group, an S3 may reflect exclusively the rapid diastolic filling rate and high stroke volume typical of these conditions even in a setting of compensated left ventricular performance.

380. Ishmail AA, Wing S, Ferguson J, et al. Interobserver agreement by auscultation in the presence of a third heart sound in patients with congestive heart failure. *Chest.* 1987;91:870-3.

Discusses how in 81 patients admitted to a cardiology ward, there was poor agreement among four observers (an internist, a medical resident, a cardiologist, and a cardiology fellow) for the presence of S3. Cumulative kappa was 0.4 for the entire group of patients, 0.3 for those with heart failure, and 0.1 for those without it. This paper, although not intended to ascertain the presence or absence of S3, raises questions about its use in practice. Fortunately for those of us who believe in the science of physical examination, not all series mirror these results (*see* reference 403).

381. Spodick DH, Quarry-Piggott VM. Fourth heart sound as a normal finding in older persons. *N Engl J Med.* 1973;288:140-1.

Some of the groundwork supporting the study of Benchimol (*see* reference 378).

382. Stapleton JF. The third heart sound of heart failure: valuable only when heard. *Chest.* 1987;91:801-2.

A third sound is meaningful although not always pathologic. The absence of an audible S3 does not permit any inference about the absence of heart failure.

383. Timmis AJ. The third heart sound [Editorial]. *Br Med J.* **1987;294:326-7.**

Very short editorial summarizing recent insights.

384. Vine DL. Galloping disagreement. *Kans Med.* 1995;96(1):38-9.

A disagreeable recounting of others' studies showing poor agreement in detection of both S3 and S4. The author wonders whether better reproducibility would shorten hospital stays. It is true that examination must earn its keep, but we believe that nihilism is no remedy.

385. Wilken MK, Meyers DG, Laski PA, et al. Mechanism of disappearance of S3 with maturation. *Am J Cardiol.* **1989;64:1394-6.**

Cross-sectional study suggesting that S3 disappears with maturation due to a decrease and slowing of early diastolic left ventricular filling caused by the age-related increase in left ventricular mass.

Murmurs

386. Aronow WS, Kronzon I. Prevalence and severity of valvular aortic stenosis determined by Doppler echocardiography and its association with echocardiographic and electrocardiographic left ventricular hypertrophy and physical signs of aortic stenosis in elderly patients. *Am J Cardiol.* **1991;67:776-7.**

Discusses how classic features of severity in aortic stenosis (late, prolonged murmur, delayed carotid upstrokes, decreased A2 intensity) increase in frequency as echocardiographic severity increases but are not specific enough to be clinically definitively discriminating (*see also* reference 400).

387. Forsell G, Jonasson R, Orinius E. Identifying severe aortic valvular stenosis by bedside examination. *Acta Med Scand.* 1985;218:397-400.

Severe aortic stenosis can be effectively predicted by the presence of a mid-systolic (rather than early systolic) peak of the intensity of the murmur. These results must be analyzed with caution, keeping Aronow's data in perspective.

Aronow's older work on the subject is also worth reading:

388. Aronow WS, Kronzon I. Correlation of prevalence and severity of valvular aortic stenosis determined by continuous-wave Doppler echocardiography with physical signs of aortic stenosis in patients aged 62 to 100 years with aortic systolic ejection murmurs. *Am J Cardiol.* 1987;60:399-401.

As in other studies, murmur characteristics do not satisfactorily predict hemodynamics or even the diagnosis of aortic stenosis.

389. Burch GE, Phillips JH. Murmurs of aortic stenosis and mitral insufficiency masquerading as one another. *Am Heart J.* 1963;66:439-42.

Early review, before echocardiography and other modern diagnostic techniques, acknowledging multiple confusing auscultatory features whereby the examiner can infer the wrong valve lesion, the absence of the actual one, or multiple lesions when a unitary pathology is responsible.

390. Cotter L, Logan RL, Poole A. Innocent systolic murmurs in healthy 40-year-old men. *J R Coll Physicians Lond.* 1980;14:128-9.

In this study, 16% of the cohort had soft systolic murmurs, mostly at the lower left sternal border, without heart disease. Innocent systolic murmurs may first appear in adulthood.

391. Fraser AG, Weston CF. The Graham Steell murmur: eponymous serendipity? *J R Coll Physicians Lond.* 1991;25:66-70.

Some illuminating medical history about a murmur that is commonly mistaken for aortic insufficiency.

392. Hegde BM. Auscultation for mitral valve prolapse [Letter]. *Lancet.* 1994;344:1446.

Asserts that the knee-chest position brings out the click and murmur and is easily assumed by the typically young and mobile patient in whom the diagnosis is suspected but not confirmed by conventional cardiac auscultation.

393. Kinney EL. Causes of false-negative auscultation of regurgitant lesions: a Doppler echocardiographic study of 294 patients. *J Gen Intern Med.* 1988;3:429-34.

Discusses application of pulsed Doppler study to the investigation of clinical puzzles. Concludes that the sensitivity of auscultation is poor but the specificity is high, apropos valvular insufficiency.

394. Lembo NJ, Dell'Italia LJ, Crawford MH, O'Rourke RA. Bedside diagnosis of systolic murmurs. *N Engl J Med.* 1988;318:1572-8.

Analysis of the predictive value of various manipulative phenomena, in a highly defined group. Readers must heed the authors' caveat about extending the findings to unselected patients pending large parallel series in other groups such as elderly outpatients, but the importance and conclusiveness of the assertions within the limits that the authors specify are impressive. Essential reading.

395. Olive KE, Grassman ED. Mitral valve prolapse: comparison of diagnosis by physical examination and echocardiography. *South Med J.* 1990;93:1266-9.

Discussion of how if a systolic click and murmur are heard, mitral prolapse will be found on echocardiogram two thirds of the time—and one third of studies will be normal! Other combinations of findings have less predictive value.

396. **Spodick DH, Kerigan AT, de la Paz LR, et al. Clavicular auscultation: preferential clavicular transmission and amplification of aortic valve murmurs.** *Chest.* **1976;70:337-40.**

In a small study, 12 of 14 patients with aortic valvular murmurs had amplification over the clavicle, in contrast to the usually described attenuation over the carotid.

397. **Wei JY, Fortuin NJ. Diastolic sounds and murmurs associated with mitral valve prolapse.** *Circulation.* **1981;63:559-64.**

Discusses how diastolic sounds are heard in a small proportion of patients with mitral valve prolapse. An early diastolic sound seems to coincide with the recoaptation of the mitral leaflets. An early diastolic murmur may also be present and possibly represents a continuation of the late systolic murmur during isovolumic relaxation, when a pressure gradient is still present between the left atrium and the left ventricle.

Special settings and specific conditions

398. **Abbas F, Sapira JD. Mayne's sign is not pathognomonic of aortic insufficiency.** *South Med J.* **1987;80:1051-2.**

One of the old signs in the attic that belongs in the trash bin, not restored to practice.

399. **Aronow WS, Kronzon I. Correlation of prevalence and severity of aortic regurgitation detected by pulsed Doppler echocardiography with the murmur of aortic regurgitation in elderly patients in a long-term health care facility.** *Am J Cardiol.* **1989;63:128-9.**

The most striking observation is not the technologic correlate, but the presence of a diastolic murmur in 25.1% of an unselected group of nursing home patients, a figure exceeding the prevalence reported by others by at least an order of magnitude.

400. **Lombard JT, Selzer A. Valvular aortic stenosis: a clinical and hemodynamic profile of patients.** *Ann Intern Med.* **1987;106:292-8.**

Particularly in elderly persons, the old familiar signs are often lacking, even in tight aortic stenosis as defined by left-heart catheterization. Lesser murmur intensity, normal pulse pressure, and preserved carotid upstroke do not exclude this condition.

401. **Sapira JD. Quincke, de Musset, Duroziez, and Hill: some aortic regurgitations.** *South Med J.* 1981;74:459-67.

Consideration of these four peripheral signs in terms of their modern application and predictive values, which render them unworthy of continued use.

Prosthetic valves

402. **Smith ND, Raizada V, Abrams J. Auscultation of the normally functioning prosthetic valve.** *Ann Intern Med.* 1981;95:594-8.

There is relief for examiners confused by the noises that these devices create.

Heart failure

403. **Butman SM, Ewy GA, Standen JR, et al. Bedside cardiovascular examination in patients with severe chronic heart failure: importance of rest or inducible jugular venous distension.** *J Am Coll Cardiol.* 1993; 22:968-74.

See combined review in reference 412.

404. **Chakko S, Woska D, Martinez H, et al. Clinical, radiographic, and hemodynamic correlations in chronic congestive heart failure: conflicting results may lead to inappropriate care.** *Am J Med.* 1991; 90:353-9.

See combined review in reference 412.

405. **Clausen JL. CHF, rales and the Dco [Editorial].** *Chest.* 1990;98:523-4.

Discusses how in chronic congestive heart failure, the presence of crackles is a strong predictor of a decreased diffusing capacity for carbon monoxide (Dco). If there is congestive heart failure without crackles, but with a decreased Dco, a second cause for the low diffusing capacity must be sought.

406. **Deguchi F, Hirakawa S, Gotoh K, et al. Prognostic significance of posturally induced crackles: long-term follow-up of patients after recovery from acute myocardial infarction.** *Chest.* 1993;103;1457-62.

Describes how crackles induced by postural changes or leg elevation 3 to 4 weeks after a myocardial infarction were used to predict an increase in late mortality beyond differences in hemodynamics or left ventricular function. The results are intriguing, but methodologic constraints demand corroboration of results before they can be accepted.

407. Liebson PR, Klein LW. A primer on LV assessment. Part 1: History and physical examination: clinical symptoms may not reflect the extent of the disorder. *J Crit Illness.* 1996;11(5):281-8.

A useful source for the medical student on the initial approach to clinical manifestations of left ventricular dysfunction. Does not cover global cardiac assessment.

408. Marantz PR, Kaplan MC, Alderman MH. Clinical diagnosis of congestive heart failure in patients with acute dyspnea. *Chest.* 1990;97:776-81.

Describes how in patients older than 40 years presenting to the emergency room with dyspnea, the abdominojugular test and the blood pressure response to the Valsalva maneuver were valid in the diagnosis of heart failure. However, their use did not add substantially to the overall clinician's assessment.

409. Marantz PR, Tobin JN, Wassertheil-Smoller S, et al. The relationship between left ventricular systolic function and congestive heart failure diagnosed by clinical criteria. *Circulation.* 1988;77:607-12.

See combined review in reference 412.

410. Poole-Wilson PA. The origin of symptoms in patients with chronic heart failure. *Eur Heart J.* 1988;9(Suppl H):49-53.

Review article that, although not exhaustive, discusses evidence for the lack of association between symptoms and central hemodynamics in chronic congestive heart failure.

411. Siegel JL, Miller A, Brown KL, et al. Pulmonary diffusing capacity in left ventricular dysfunction. *Chest.* 1990;98:550-3.

See combined review in reference 405.

412. Stevenson LW, Perloff JK. The limited reliability of physical signs for estimating hemodynamics in chronic heart failure. *JAMA.* 1989; 261:884-8.

These articles (references 403, 404, 409, and 412) substantiate the concept of poor predictability of central hemodynamics and cardiac performance by physical diagnosis alone, and the need for technologic measurement of such variables. However, each has its own unique features and particular results that may be applied in practice. For example, Stevenson and Perloff show the value of the proportional pulse pressure defined as [SBP-DBP]/SBP (i.e., pulse pressure/SBP) in estimating cardiac index: if less than 0.25, 91% of patients had a cardiac index of less than 2.2 L/min. In addition, Butman and colleagues (reference 403) show, in their excellent paper, that the presence of jugular venous distension or a positive abdominojugular test indicated a probability of 86% that the pulmonary capillary wedge pressure exceeded 18 mm Hg.

413. **Wilson JR, Rayos G, Yeoh TK, et al. Dissociation between exertional symptoms and circulatory function in patients with heart failure.** *Circulation.* **1995;92:47-53.**

State-of-the-art methods, including use of pulmonary artery catheters in the treadmill laboratory, are employed in this study to demonstrate the lack of relationship between exertional symptoms and the degree of hemodynamic dysfunction in 82 patients with chronic congestive heart failure. Such observations attest to the existence of other nonhemodynamic determinants of functional capacity in heart failure, probably both physical and emotional.

Ischemic heart disease

414. **Craddock LD. The physical examination in acute ischemic syndromes.** *J Emerg Med.* **1991;9:55-60.**

Discusses how physical examination has minimal power to detect ischemia or infarction. Complications, however, may be recognized by this modality, and examination permits the all-important functional assessments of the heart and of the patient.

415. **Dell'Italia LJ, Starling MR, O'Rourke RA. Physical examination for exclusion of hemodynamically important right ventricular infarction.** *Ann Intern Med.* **1983;99:608-11.**

Extremely convincing methods support the claim that the absence of both Kussmaul's sign and elevated jugular venous pressure in a patient with acute inferior-wall myocardial infarction means that there is no major right ventricular infarction.

416. **Forrester JS, Diamond GA, Swan HJC. Correlative classification of clinical and hemodynamic function after acute myocardial infarction.** *Am J Cardiol.* **1977;39:137-45.**

A classic paper on the correlation between clinical and hemodynamic subsets in acute myocardial infarction, and their prediction of mortality. Forrester's classification remains in use in cardiac care units around the world. Mandatory reading. The inference from crackles in this setting, a legacy of the older Killip classification, remains central in bedside evaluation and monitoring today.

417. Connors AF Jr, McCaffree DR, Gray BA. Evaluation of right-heart catheterization in the critically ill patient without acute myocardial infarction. *N Engl J Med.* 1983;308:263-7.

This study is widely treated simplistically, as meaning one needs a "Swan" in nonmyocardial infarction medical intensive-care patients, because its readings so often refine the clinical impression. This seminal paper's messages are more complex and subtle.

418. Friedman M, Ghandour G. Medical diagnosis of type A behavior. *Am Heart J.* 1993;126:607-18.

Videotaped sessions with patients with previously known type A or type B personalities were used to validate a scoring system to identify type A behavior. Thirty-three manifestations of "time urgency" and "free floating hostility" were studied. Despite the controversy on the impact of type A behavior on coronary disease, this article has value in its detail and peculiarity.

Combined heart and lung disease

419. Hill NS. The cardiac exam in lung disease. *Clin Chest Med.* 1987;8:273-85.

Excellent prototype of specialized, directed examination tailored to special needs.

420. Zema MJ, Masters AP, Margouleff D. Dyspnea: the heart or the lungs? Differentiation at the bedside by use of the simple Valsalva maneuver. *Chest.* 1984;85:59-64.

An alternative to nuclide studies. It determines whether increased dyspnea in a patient with obstructive airways disease reflects the pulmonary disorder only (sinusoidal response) or left ventricular dysfunction as well (absent overshoot or square wave).

Pericardial disease

421. Flickinger AL, Peller PA, Deran BP, Burket MW. Pacemaker-induced friction rub and apical thrill. *Chest.* 1992;102:323-4.

Case report revisiting the issue of systolic sounds and murmurs generated by temporary pacemaker wires. The presence of an apical thrill without any evidence of tricuspid insufficiency suggests a potential role for vibrations of the wire against the right ventricular wall as the mechanism for such sounds.

422. Kar PM, Leehey D, Aronoff GR. Pseudo pericardial rub [Letter]. *J Ky Med Assoc.* 1992;90:528.

Alleges that friction of skin against the diaphragm of the stethoscope, confined to diastole, explains two cases in cachectic patients. The patients could not have had genuine rubs because the echocardiogram (of the one in whom it was done) was negative . . .

423. Markiewicz W, Brik A, Brook G, et al. Pericardial rub in pericardial effusion: lack of correlation with amount of fluid. *Chest.* **1980;77:643-6.**

A thoughtful investigation from the early period of echocardiography, exploding the old pearl that "larger effusions lose the rub because the surfaces are no longer in close enough apposition to rub against one another," a feature that by definition cannot be true at the reflection of layers.

424. Tyberg TI, Goodyer AV, Langou RA. Genesis of pericardial knock in constrictive pericarditis. *Am J Cardiol.* **1980;46:570-5.**

Advanced technology permits new insight into the mechanism. Accounts for cases lacking a knock.

Peripheral Vasculature

Arteries

General material

425. Crawford MH, Fowler NO. *Inspection and Palpation of Venous and Arterial Pulses.* **Dallas: American Heart Association; 1990.**

Perhaps the most unique and freestanding of the four booklets in the series "Examination of the Heart."

426. Kurtz KJ. Dynamic vascular auscultation. *Am J Med.* **1984;76:1066-74.**

Fine mixture of basic science and bedside application. However, one ought to avoid undertaking diagnostic carotid compression.

Superficial temporal arteries

427. Curran RE. Palpation of the superficial temporal artery in normal persons [Letter]. *Arch Ophthalmol.* **1986;104:1756.**

This study shows that elderly, normal persons, including those with widespread and severe atherosclerosis, seldom if ever lack a palpable pulse at this site, in contrast to those with temporal arteritis (giant cell arteritis).

Carotid arteries

428. Chambers BR, Norris JW. Outcome in patients with asymptomatic neck bruits. *N Engl J Med.* **1986;315:860-5.**

This physical finding is easier to detect than to act on. Careful statistical study leads to a usable decision tree.

429. Reed CA, Toole JF. Clinical technique for identification of external carotid bruits. *Neurology.* **1981;31:744-6.**

Asserts, based on one well-studied case, that one can attenuate a bruit originating in the external carotid artery by compressing the ipsilateral superficial temporal artery and facial artery. See analogous issues in reference 689.

430. Sauve J-S, Laupacis A, Ostbye T, et al. Does this patient have a clinically important carotid bruit? (The Rational Clinical Examination.) *JAMA*. 1993;270:2843-6.

Concise, practical review on auscultation of the carotid arteries and interpretation of findings.

431. Coyle TJ. Detection of carotid stenosis by physical examination [Letter]. *JAMA*. 1994;271:1908.

Pulsation of the central retinal artery during compression of the eye through the lid may indicate compromise of the ipsilateral carotid circulation.

432. Lubic LG. Detection of carotid stenosis by physical examination [Letter]. *JAMA*. 1994;271:1908.

Extension of a carotid bruit into diastole indicates a high degree of stenosis.

433. Laupacis A, Ostbye T, Feagan B, et al. Detection of carotid stenosis by physical examination [Letter in reply]. *JAMA*. 1994;271:1908.

Response to the two letters above, acknowledging that neither of the assertions has been formally validated.

434. Sauve J-S, Thorpe KE, Sackett DL, et al. Can bruits distinguish high-grade from moderate symptomatic carotid stenosis? *Ann Intern Med*. 1994;120:633-7.

Discusses how the presence and characteristics of cervical bruits do not have adequate power to predict the degree of carotid artery stenosis. In appropriate clinical scenarios, further investigation should not be withheld because of the absence of a bruit.

435. Van Ruiswyk J, Noble H, Sigmann P. The natural history of carotid bruits in elderly persons. *Ann Intern Med*. 1990;112:340-3.

The most intriguing finding of this study was that bruits very frequently disappeared, with no corresponding clinical event, on repeated examination 1 year after detection.

Upper limb arteries

436. Leach RM, McBrien DJ. Brachioradial delay: a new clinical indicator of the severity of aortic stenosis. *Lancet*. 1990;335:1199-201.

According to this intriguing study in a small group of patients, if the brachial and radial pulses are palpated on a single side simultaneously and a palpable delay between the two can be felt, a substantial peak transvalvular gradient is likely. Within the group, congestive heart failure from nonvalvular causes did not lead to false-positives.

437. **Martyn CN, Frier BM, Corrall RJ, et al. Why palpate the radial artery?** *Lancet.* **1981;1:89-90.**

Autopsy correlation that would appear to disagree with the implications of the Osler maneuver (*see* reference 132).

438. **O'Mara K, Sullivan B. A simple bedside test to identify ulnar collateral flow [Letter].** *Ann Intern Med.* **1995;123:637.**

Describes an analogue to the Allen test. It uses the reading from a pulse oximeter as the marker of effective flow. The authors recommend its use in patients with peripheral hypoperfusion. Unfortunately, no data are presented comparing its efficacy to the older Allen test, which does not require the expensive technology of pulse oximetry at the bedside.

439. Kruse JA. Use of pulse oximetry for assessing ulnar collateral flow [Letter]. *Ann Intern Med.* 1996;125:522.

Evidence against the utility of the above method, drawing on additional investigations and basic science work.

440. O'Mara K. Use of pulse oximetry for assessing ulnar collateral flow [Letter in reply]. *Ann Intern Med.* 1996;125:522.

Argues that the ordinary Allen test is too restrictive, and acknowledges that some patient groups will be unsuitable for this new test.

Aorta

441. **Beede SD, Ballard DJ, James EM, et al. Positive predictive value of clinical suspicion of abdominal aortic aneurysm: implications for efficient use of abdominal ultrasonography.** *Arch Intern Med.* **1990;150:549-51.**

Careful analysis by a researcher trained in clinical epidemiology, who untangles a series of problems relating to screening, false-positive examinations in thin normal persons with pulsatile aortas, and so on.

442. **Cole CW, Barber GG, Bouchard AG, et al. Abdominal aortic aneurysm: consequences of a positive family history.** *Can J Surg.* **1989;32:117-20.**

Describes how siblings of patients, particularly if the patient's parent or another sibling was also affected, have a large incremental risk compared with controls.

443. **Guarino JR. Abdominal aortic aneurysm: a new diagnostic sign.** *J Kansas Med Soc.* **1975;76(5):108, 15A.**

Discussion of an additional sign: mobility side-to-side versus craniocaudal fixation helps to define the mass as aortic.

444. **Lederle FA, Walker JM, Reinke DB. Selective screening for abdominal aortic aneurysms with physical examination and ultrasound.** *Arch Intern Med.* **1988;148:1753-6.**

Describes how for patients with a waist 100 cm (40 inches) or greater, aneurysms are unlikely to be felt even if large, and ultrasonography becomes a more appropriate screening test. For thin patients, palpation works well.

Lower limb arteries

445. **Brearley S, Shearman CP, Simms MH. Peripheral pulse palpation: an unreliable physical sign.** *Ann R Coll Surg Engl.* **1992;74(3):169-71.**

Foot pulses are sometimes reported to be present when they are absent, according to a reference standard of examination by two vascular surgeons. It is better known that foot pulses are also frequently missed when they are present. This particular study is weakened by the tiny number of patients and immense number of examinations performed during a short timespan on each, which might lead to local edema or vasospasm—vitiating results.

446. **Christensen JH, Freundlich M, Jacobsen BA, Falstie-Jensen N. Clinical relevance of pedal pulse palpation in patients suspected of peripheral arterial insufficiency.** *J Intern Med.* **1989;226:95-9.**

Absent foot pulses with normal warm skin are a combination geriatricians learn to ignore. This article addresses the assessment of ischemic ulcers apropos healing: palpable pulses augur a better outcome in this setting. Provides several conclusions, which are not all equally supported by the data.

447. **Insall RL, Davies RJ, Prout WG. Significance of Buerger's test in the assessment of lower limb ischaemia.** *J R Soc Med.* **1989;82:729-31.**

Describes how in persons with severe claudication, pallor on elevation and a flush of dependent rubor are correlated with more severe and more distal arterial stenoses.

448. **Magee TR, Stanley PR, al Mufti R, et al. Should we palpate foot pulses?** *Ann R Coll Surg Engl.* **1992;74(3):166-8.**

When palpation is performed, the absence or presence of the dorsalis pedis pulse is more consistently agreed upon by examiners of widely varying experience than is that of the posterior tibial. (With the posterior tibial, by the way, the opposite is true—i.e., the results are more consistent when the Doppler probe is used.) Contests the notion that the thickened walls of pedal arteries in persons with widespread severe atheromatous vascular disease affecting multiple organs disable pulse palpation in them.

449. Dormandy JA. Palpation of peripheral pulses: a difficult art [Editorial]. *Ann R Coll Surg Engl.* 1992;74(3):155.

A short comment on reference 448 and on the paper by Brearley and associates (reference 445). Mentions the harm and hazard in fabricating a pulse where none is present. Reminds us that Doppler systolic pressure recording is neither as easy nor as reliable as we might wish. The arguments miss one key point—namely, that elderly persons in whom no pulse can be palpated often have adequate perfusion as judged by lack of claudication and of ulcers.

450. Mozes M, Mozes MF. Gastrocnemius compression sign in arterial insufficiency of the leg. *J Cardiovasc Surg.* 1987;28:277-8.

Proposes unifying mechanisms for positive findings (tenderness on squeezing the calf with two hands) in both arterial and venous insufficiency.

451. O'Sullivan J, Bain H. Differential collapsing pulses: a new clinical sign [Letter]. *Ann Intern Med.* 1993;119:540.

Discusses how a collapsing pulse in the lower extremities with normal upper extremity pulses may be a clue to pulmonic regurgitation in patients with complex congenital heart disease consisting of an interrupted aortic arch and a single ventricle. Rarest zebra in this book.

Veins

Neck veins

452. Cook DJ, Simel DL. Does this patient have abnormal central venous pressure? (The Rational Clinical Examination.) *JAMA.* 1996; 275:630-4.

Heroic handling of a difficult topic. Advocates the use of the right *internal* jugular waveform and speaks of recognizing a meniscus on it, an oxymoron. Suggests specifying the jugular venous pressure rather than adding 5 cm and speaking of the ECVP (estimated central venous pressure), a term that we consider less subject to misinterpretation. Pragmatic, perspicacious description of optimal technique for inspecting the veins and conducting the abdominojugular test, but does not recognize its correlation with left heart dysfunction (*see* reference 453).

453. Ewy GA. The abdominojugular test: technique and hemodynamic correlates. *Ann Intern Med.* 1988;109:456-60.

Concise, understandable insights on this old test, widely called the hepatojugular reflux test (or, erroneously, the hepatojugular reflex). The data on elevated pulmonary capillary pressure—that is, *left* heart implications—will be new to many readers.

454. Ewy GA. Evaluation of the neck veins. *Hosp Pract.* **(March 30). 1987; 22(3A):72-5, 79-80.**

A simple review demystifying the examination of the neck veins. Two important drawbacks: the use of abdominal compression is mentioned but not discussed and there are no references.

455. Meyer TE, Sareli P, Marcus RH, et al. Mechanism underlying Kussmaul's sign in chronic constrictive pericarditis. *Am J Cardiol.* **1989; 64:1069-72.**

Intensive and probing investigation of the mechanism and meaning of the sign in two patients, with a bit of discussion about the sign in general.

456.   Schneiderman H. More questions on Kussmaul's sign [Letter]. *Am J Cardiol.* 1990;66:772.
See combined review in reference 457.

457.   Meyer TE, McGregor M. More questions on Kussmaul's sign [Reply]. *Am J Cardiol.* 1990; 66:772.
Some questions remain unanswerable. Unfortunately, other questions addressed in the inquiry are not even tackled in the response.

Abdomen

General material

458. Levitt RE, Roth JL. General physical examination. In: Berk JE, Haubrich WS, Kalser MH, et al, eds. *Bockus Gastroenterology*. 4th ed. Philadelphia: WB Saunders; 1985;1:257-75.

Although the newer edition (5th ed., 1994) of the Bockus multivolume text has a good initial chapter on the history and examination by SC Wolf, it does not supplant the old standard by Levitt and Roth. The latter contains some errors and some dated material, such as a segment on asthenic and hypersthenic habitus. Nevertheless, the chapter in the earlier edition of the book offers a wealth of insight on the whole-body examination as viewed from a gastroenterologic perspective. Contains the only account of the timing of esophageal transit at the bedside that we can find anywhere.

459. Mellinkoff SM. "Stethoscope sign" [Letter]. *N Engl J Med*. 1964; 271:630.

See combined review in reference 460.

460. Meyerowitz BR. Abdominal palpation by stethoscope [Letter]. *Arch Surg*. 1976;111:831.

Discusses how patients who exaggerate tenderness can be identified and better examined at the same time.

461. Oldstone MB. Stethoscopic treachery [Letter]. *N Engl J Med*. 1965;272:107.

Describes a striking, false-positive stethoscope sign in a patient who had purulent peritonitis. The need for serial observation is stressed.

462. Neumann MJ, Meyer CT, Dutton JL, Smith R. Hold that x-ray: aspirate pH and auscultation prove enteral tube placement. *J Clin Gastroenterol*. 1995;20:293-5.

Discusses trying to omit a radiograph to check placement of a Dobhoff-weighted enteral feeding tube. Auscultation erroneously suggested proper gastric placement in 15 of 16 instances of misplaced tubes. A pH of aspirated fluid less than 4, taken without confounding food in the stomach, allowed one to dispense with the radiograph. A pH greater than 4 is more difficult to interpret, particularly when the patient is receiving antipeptic medications. For another view, *see* reference 463.

463. Metheny N, McSweeney M, Wehrle MA, Wiersma L. Effectiveness of the auscultatory method in predicting feeding tube location. *Nursing Res.* 1990;39:262-7.

Discusses how auscultation is inadequate to predict the location of soft nasoenteric feeding tubes. Both accuracy and inter-rater agreement were not dissimilar to results expected from chance alone.

464. Priebe WM, DaCosta LR, Beck IT. Is epigastric tenderness a sign of peptic ulcer disease? *Gastroenterology.* **1982;82:16-9.**

A discussion of how epigastric tenderness on palpation, although quite reproducible, is a poor test to predict peptic ulcer disease or any esophagogastroduodenal disease.

History

465. Payne JE. Symptoms and the diagnosis of bowel cancer: a critical view. *Med J Aust.* **1988;148:505-7.**

Addresses the issue of who needs colonoscopy. Discusses major difficulties with the insensitivity and notorious nonspecificity of symptoms as guides for investigation for colon cancer. Makes more of recent-onset symptoms in the age group at greatest risk.

466. Talley NJ, Phillips SF, Melton LJ III, et al. A patient questionnaire to identify bowel disease. *Ann Intern Med.* **1989;111:671-4.**

Although the central points of this article are well taken, some of the side-lights are even more interesting. For example, pain that awakens one from sleep, long considered grave, was present in most patients with irritable bowel syndrome and nonulcer dyspepsia and in 4% of normal patients.

467. Drossman DA. A questionnaire for functional bowel disorders. *Ann Intern Med.* 1989;111:627-9.

Excellent accompanying editorial that makes one want to read and use Talley's paper.

Acute abdomen

468. Aldea PA, Meehan JP, Sternbach G. The acute abdomen and Murphy's signs. *J Emerg Med.* **1986;4:57-63.**

Reviews much history of medicine, including the original papers, and thereby dispels some of the murk—including that about the two separate Murphy signs.

469. Arnbjornsson E, Bengmark S. Auscultation of bowel sounds in patients with suspected acute appendicitis—an aid in the diagnosis? *Eur Surg Res.* **1983;15:24-7.**

Study with substantial methodologic limitations (sample size, control group, equipment) that nonetheless shows that there may be a lateralization in the decrease of bowel sounds. Right-sided sounds become fainter than left-sided sounds in appendicitis, more noticeably in the intermediate stages of the disease.

470. Bennett DH, Tambeur LJMT, Campbell WB. Use of coughing test to diagnose peritonitis. *BMJ.* **1994;308:1336.**

Discusses the sensitivity (78%) and specificity (79%) of coughing to detect peritoneal irritation without the occasional cruelty of rebound testing.

471. Gray DW, Dixon JM, Collin J. The closed eyes sign: an aid to diagnosing non-specific abdominal pain. *Br Med J.* **1988;297:837.**

Demonstrates how patients who do not vigilantly watch the examiner are more likely, although not certain, to have no acute surgical cause of their pain.

472. Collin J, Gray DW. The eyes closed sign. *Br Med J.* 1987;295:1656.

An original, short description that was part of the underpinning of the longer and more definitive paper (*see* reference 471).

473. Odom NJ. Facial expression in acute appendicitis. *Ann R Coll Surg Engl.* **1982;64:260-1.**

Discusses an aura of malaise that is not the same as wincing. This article is devoid of any scientific commitment. In desperate need of a prospective blinded study, which could very easily be accomplished with photographs made before operative or conservative management, then compared with the final diagnosis.

474. Silen W. *Cope's Early Diagnosis of the Acute Abdomen.* **19th ed. New York: Oxford University Press; 1996.**

Establishes the continuing primacy of bedside assessment over all laboratory tests and imaging results persists in this archetypical problem requiring expert interview and examination.

475. Thomson WH, Francis DM. Abdominal-wall tenderness: a useful sign in the acute abdomen. *Lancet.* **1977;2:1053-4.**

An update on an old sign, surprisingly little recognized: a sit-up equivalent tenses the abdominal wall; if the tenderness is not thereby reduced, its source may lie in the abdominal wall rather than intraperitoneally. Unfortunately, intraperitoneal inflammation can spread to the abdominal musculature and produce false reassurance that the source of the tenderness lies in the abdominal wall.

Cullen's sign and variants in acute abdomen

476. **Chung MA, Oung CO, Szilagyi A. Cullen's sign: it doesn't always mean hemorrhagic pancreatitis.** *Am J Gastroenterol.* **1992;87:1026-8.**

Discusses how the Cullen sign occurred in a patient with spontaneous splenic rupture from mononucleosis: an additional item on a long list of non-pancreatitic causes.

477. **Cullen TS. A new sign in ruptured extrauterine pregnancy.** *Am J Obstet.* **1918;7:457.**

Cullen's account of his sign, due to an ectopic pregnancy. How the sign came to be strongly associated with pancreatitis is not clear.

478. **Grey Turner G. Local discoloration of the abdominal wall as a sign of acute pancreatitis.** *Br J Surg.* **1920;7:394-5.**

Grey Turner's landmark description of his sign.

479. **Meyers MA, Feldberg MAM, Oliphant M. Grey Turner's sign and Cullen's sign in acute pancreatitis.** *Gastrointest Radiol.* **1989;14:31-7.**

Shows that these two signs occur in less than 3% of cases of pancreatitis, perhaps because of the specific tissue and fascial planes that blood and secretions need to track around to produce the signs.

Ascites

480. **Cattau EL Jr, Benjamin SB, Knuff TE, Castell DO. The accuracy of the physical examination in the diagnosis of suspected ascites.** *JAMA.* **1982;247:1164-6.**

Describes work with patients on the borderline. Meticulous clinical methodology and statistical analysis show that no individual sign possesses satisfactory accuracy, nor does any combination of signs.

481. **Cummings S, Papadakis M, Melnick J, et al. The predictive value of physical examinations for ascites.** *West J Med.* **1985;142:633-6.**

Prototype of modern bedside diagnostic research. Statistical analysis and a review of cases studied by ultrasonography show that patients with a prolonged prothrombin time *and* a positive fluid wave are almost certain to have ascites and do not need to have ultrasonography.

482. Simel DL, Halvorsen RA Jr, Feussner JR. Quantitating bedside diagnosis: clinical evaluation of ascites. *J Gen Intern Med.* 1988;3:423-8.

Careful evaluation of operating characteristics of different aspects of history and examination in the identification of ascites. In addition, results show that, based on overall impressions, clinicians are quite good at predicting the presence but not the absence of ascites.

483. Williams JW Jr, Simel DL. Does this patient have ascites? How to divine fluid in the abdomen. (The Rational Clinical Examination.) *JAMA.* 1992;267:2645-8.

Overview of the clinical features of ascites, with focus on discriminating statistics. A very useful article.

Chronic abdominal symptoms

484. Fielding JF. The right iliac fossa squelch sign: a marker of the irritable bowel syndrome. *J Clin Gastroenterol.* 1981;3:25-6.

Discusses how on palpating the cecum in the right iliac fossa, the colon is excessively palpable and there is "a sensation akin to a fine deep-seated surgical emphysema nearly always accompanied by a squelching sound." The same sign is found more widespread in the abdomen in some cases of regional enteritis, but when confined to the right iliac fossa, it seems to indicate irritable bowel syndrome. Variants of the sign have been noted and have been considered difficult to describe for more than a century. Fielding has described other features of this syndrome that are worth considering (references 485–487).

485. Fielding JF. Clinical and radiological manifestations of the irritable bowel syndrome. *J Irish Coll Phys Surg.* 1978;8:11-5.

A short compendium, with specific features not listed in the other papers.

486. Fielding JF. Detailed history and examination assist positive clinical diagnosis of the irritable bowel syndrome. *J Clin Gastroenterol.* 1983;5:495-7.

The recognition of manner that is inappropriate to content in giving a history, as described by the author, should be engrafted upon us all.

487. Fielding JF. Per rectum examination in the irritable bowel syndrome. *J Irish Med Assoc.* 1979;72:200-2.

Describes a special variant tenderness on rectal mucosal "tap" by examiner's finger. This is more characteristic of persons with this syndrome than of other persons.

488. Gallegos NC, Hobsley M. Recognition and treatment of abdominal wall pain. *J R Soc Med.* 1989;82:343-4.

Discusses how if the picture accords with an abdominal wall source, a diagnostic trial of local anesthetic injection may secure the impression and relieve the problem simultaneously.

489. Gray DW, Dixon JM, Seabrook G, Collin J. Is abdominal wall tenderness a useful sign in the diagnosis of non-specific abdominal pain? *Ann R Coll Surg Engl.* 1988;70:233-4.

Followup to Thomson's earlier work cited in reference 475, with similar conclusions but also some caution.

490. Thomson WH, Dawes RF, Carter SS. Abdominal wall tenderness: a useful sign in chronic abdominal pain. *Br J Surg.* 1991;78:223-5.

Describes how, as in the acute abdomen (*see* reference 475), a positive sign predicts the absence of intraperitoneal disease.

Kidneys and renal vasculature

491. Eipper DF, Gifford RW Jr, Stewart BH, et al. Abdominal bruits in renovascular hypertension. *Am J Cardiol.* 1976;37:48-52.

Descriptive study of characteristics of renal arterial bruits. A combined systolic-diastolic bruit, present in up to three-fourths of patients with fibromuscular dysplasia of the renal artery, confers a high likelihood of response to revascularization.

492. O'Reilly S, Keogh JAB. Palpating enlarged kidneys. *Ir Med J.* 1992; 85(3):89.

Recommends that the examiner have the patient lie supine on a hard surface, then place one hand in the costovertebral angle and at end-inspiration push the other hand firmly and deeply below the costal margin—presumably posterior to the liver edge—to trap the kidney. They then assert that "[t]he size, consistency and shape of the organ as it slips [upward] into its normal position can be assessed." The material on percussing the kidney is not convincing.

493. Svetkey LP, Helms MJ, Dunnick NR, Klotman PE. Clinical characteristics useful in screening for renovascular disease. *South Med J.* 1990; 83:743-7.

In this study, the presence of a bruit increased the odds of renal artery stenosis elevenfold. Its sensitivity, however, was only 55%. Of features in the history, only the presence of refractory hypertension (odds ratio of 5.5) and a recent increase in the severity of hypertension (odds ratio of 2.9) had some predictive ability. Even these showed limited clinical value.

494. Turnbull JM. Is listening for abdominal bruits useful in the evaluation of hypertension? (The Rational Clinical Examination.) *JAMA*. 1995; 274:1299-301.

Discusses how high prevalence of innocent systolic abdominal bruits in normal persons, particularly young adults, makes this unsuitable as an unselected screening test. However, in persons with hypertension, particularly when the bruit extends into diastole, the predictive value is considerable and warrants further investigation. There is no need to characterize pitch, intensity, or laterality. Another fine component of the Rational Clinical Examination series.

495. Walzer A, Koenigsberg M. Examining the anterior right kidney: frequent lack of appreciation in examination of the right upper quadrant. *JAMA*. 1979;242:2320-1.

Although it focuses on diagnosis using ultrasonography, this article reminds us that the ptotic kidney can lie just beneath the surface.

Liver, gallbladder, biliary tree, jaundice

496. Callahan CW Jr. Simultaneous percussion auscultation technique for the determination of liver span. *Arch Pediatr Adolesc Med*. 1994;148:873-5.

In this study, direct percussion with simultaneous auscultation of the liver correlated very well ($r = 0.87$) with ultrasonography in the estimation of liver span. A striking contrast to McGee's statement (*see* reference 25) that auscultatory percussion is ineffective.

497. Fuller GN, Hargreaves MR, King DM. Scratch test in clinical examination of liver [Letter]. *Lancet*. 1988;1:181.

Brief note. Reports better correlation with size as determined by imaging studies than do previous studies. Proposes explanation relating to a modified technique.

498. Gilbert VE. Detection of the liver below the costal margin: comparative value of palpation, light percussion, and auscultatory percussion. *Southern Med J*. 1994;87:182-6.
Weak descriptive study: anecdote, not insight. More useful to read reference 496 or 497.

499. Meidl EJ, Ende J. Evaluation of liver size by physical examination. *J Gen Intern Med*. 1993;8:635-7.

Clear listing of the wealth of discordant data on the topic. However, the authors do not offer insight on the papers, and too many questions are not only left unanswered but are also not grappled with.

500. Michie C, Alu S, Wild K, et al. Should we estimate liver span in the right mid-clavicular line or the midline? *J Paediatr Child Health.* 1995;31:241-4.

A study in children younger than age 5 years; advocates midline for this group but acknowledges nonapplicability of this landmark to adults.

501. Naylor CD. Physical examination of the liver. (The Rational Clinical Examination.) *JAMA.* 1994;271:1859-65.

Appropriately conservative and evidence-based recommendations for what to do when performing a physical examination of the liver and how to get better at it. Discusses not only spans, palpation, and percussion but also bruits, hums, pulsation, and texture. Well centered on the clinical care of patients rather than roundsmanship.

502. Sapira JD, Williamson DL. How big is the normal liver? *Arch Intern Med.* 1979;139:971-3.

A comment on the difficulty in determining reference ranges and individual spans.

503. Sherlock S, Summerfield JA. *Color Atlas of Liver Disease*. Chicago: Year Book; 1979.

Covers examination of the liver and a host of other signs in disorders of the liver and associated organs. Memorable pictures. Superb pathologic correlation enhances the scientific validity.

504. Sherman HI, Hardison JE. The importance of a coexistent hepatic rub and bruit: a clue to the diagnosis of cancer in the liver. *JAMA.* 1979;241:1495.

The combination possesses better specificity than does either sign alone.

505. Sullivan S, Krasner N, Williams R. The clinical estimation of liver size: a comparison of techniques and an analysis of the source of error. *Br Med J.* 1976;2:1042-3.

Discusses how most signs, including the scratch test, show no consistent relation to actual liver tissue extent. Nor is scintigraphy faultless.

506. Verghese A, Dison C, Berk SL. Courvoisier's "law": an eponym in evolution. *Am J Gastroenterol.* 1987;82:248-50.

Historical review and examination of the current status of the enlarged gallbladder in a jaundiced patient (whether discovered at bedside or by other means), which can be interpreted as reflecting sustained high ductal pressure from cancer, stones, or some other cause.

507. Zoli M, Magalotti D, Grimaldi M, et al. Physical examination of the liver: is it still worth it? *Am J Gastroenterol.* **1995;90:1428-32.**

Two phrases betray bias: "The whole problem of physical measurement of liver span has become obsolete since ultrasound allowed a precise, unbiased measurement," and "The lack of accurate training in physical examination is common in Italy, and it may be the same everywhere in the world."

Spleen

508. Grover SA, Barkun AN, Sackett DL. Does this patient have spleno-megaly? (The Rational Clinical Examination.) *JAMA.* **1993;270:2218-21.**

Fantastic analytic review of splenomegaly. Must be read by any clinician who examines abdomens.

509. Barkun AN, Camus M, Green L, et al. The bedside assessment of splenic enlargement. *Am J Med.* 1991;91:512-8.

Methodologically strong article demonstrating the value of combined percussion and palpation of the spleen to identify splenomegaly. Best yield of palpation occurs in patients with abnormal percussion findings.

510. Barkun AN, Camus M, Meagher T, et al. Splenic enlargement and Traube's space: how useful is percussion? *Am J Med.* 1989;87:562-6.

Discusses how percussion gives helpful information but cannot stand alone. Careful scientific study shows what the sign can and cannot predict.

511. Hegde BM. How to detect early splenic enlargement. *Practitioner.* **1985;229:857.**

Recommends that the examiner move to the "forbidden" left side of the patient and hook the fingers around the ribs, with the patient assuming a right lateral decubitus position. The similar (but untilted) maneuver for the liver is better known.

512. Sullivan S, Williams R. Reliability of clinical techniques for detecting splenic enlargement. *Br Med J.* **1976;2:1043-4.**

A very brief note that covers several variations of palpation and percussion.

513. Tamayo SG, Rickman LS, Mathews WC, et al. Examiner dependence on physical diagnostic tests for the detection of splenomegaly: a prospective study with multiple observers. *J Gen Intern Med.* **1993;8:69-75.**

Although the methodology is very careful, the results of this study are vitiated by the small number of patients having ultrasonographically confirmed splenomegaly and by failure to separate out minimal splenomegaly undetectable by physical examination from more significant enlargement of the spleen.

514. **Yang JC, Rickman LS, Bosser SK. The clinical diagnosis of spleno-megaly.** *West J Med.* **1991;155:47-52.**

Considers physical examination and imaging studies as two means to a sin-gle end—namely, diagnosis—not as entities in competition. Reviews various methods used for the diagnosis at the bedside.

Urinary bladder

515. **Ashby EC. Detecting bladder fullness by subjective palpation.** *Lancet.* **1977;2:936-7.**

Describes how a patient may report a "call to micturition" when the clinician gently pushes one finger perpendicularly into the midline of the lower abdomen starting from above and going down stepwise toward symphysis pubis. Subject to false-positives in the anxious patient.

516. **Gardner BP, Doyle PT. Symptoms of bladder carcinoma [Letter].** *J R Coll Gen Pract.* **1987;37:367.**

Discusses how for those patients whose chief complaint is not painless hematuria, the most common complaints are urinary frequency, dysuria, and poor stream. Once infection has been treated and prostatism excluded, cases of bladder carcinoma may be detected by urinary cytology and, when indi-cated, cystoscopy.

517. **Guarino JR. Auscultatory percussion of the urinary bladder.** *Arch Intern Med.* **1985;145:1823-5.**

Describes a method that supersedes previous unsatisfactory methods and that can be used successfully even if the patient is obese or has gaseous dis-tension or ascites.

Rectum

General material

518. Dixon JM, Elton RA, Rainey JB, Macleod DAD. **Rectal examination in patients with pain in the right lower quadrant of the abdomen.** *BMJ.* 1991;302:386-8.

Purports that testing for rebound tenderness pre-empts the diagnostic yield of per rectum palpation in persons in whom acute appendicitis is suspected. Incredibly, one seventh of the large series of patients did not have a rectal examination on admission with a chief complaint of right lower quadrant abdominal pain! Central assertion is sure to provoke a firestorm of disagreement.

519. Dixon JM, Elton RA. Rectal examination in patients with abdominal pain [Letter in reply]. *BMJ.* 1991;302:1274.

Embarrassingly naive arithmetic response.

520. Eckardt VF, Kanzler G. **How reliable is digital examination for the evaluation of anal sphincter tone?** *Int J Colorectal Dis.* 1993;8:95-7.

Alleges poor correlation between manometric findings and digital assessment of sphincter pressure, despite the physical examination done by a highly experienced proctologist. However, the digital examination was performed right after manometry, and the possible confounding effect of sphincter fatigue or inadvertent dilation is not addressed. Furthermore, assessments are dichotomized into normal and abnormal, rather than viewed on a continuum. More work is needed.

521. Hennigan TW, Franks PJ, Hocken DB, Allen-Mersh TG. **Rectal examination in general practice.** *BMJ.* 1990;301:478-80.

About half of a group of British general practitioners performed fewer than five rectal examinations per month. Several catalogued reasons include patient reluctance and lack of time or of a chaperone. This article emphasizes that it is not just housestaff who seem to find every reason on earth to avoid this high-yield procedure.

522. Kemple T. Rectal examination in general practice [Letter]. *BMJ.* 1990;301:667-8.

A contentious litany that misses the point of the article.

523. Hennigan TW, Franks PJ. Rectal examination in general practice [Letter in reply]. *BMJ.* 1990;301:678.

Gently returns the focus to where it belongs, and cites a videotape on the performance of the test made by one of the authors (Dr. Allen-Mersh).

524. Hennigan TW, Franks PJ, Hocken DB, Allen-Mersh TG. Influence of undergraduate teaching on medical students' attitudes to rectal examination. *BMJ.* 1991;302:829.

Describes how the infrequency of this examination in practice, documented by this group's earlier work (*see* reference 521), relates in part to the fact that one fifth of final-year British medical students have performed fewer than ten rectal examinations.

525. Herrinton LJ, Selby JV, Friedman GD, et al. Case-control study of digital-rectal screening in relation to mortality from cancer of the distal rectum. *Am J Epidemiol.* 1995;142:961-4.

The authors claim the screening does not earn its keep in this regard, but they fail to comment on the fact that only one-fifth of the patients in both the control and cancer groups had had a screening (nonsymptom-directed) digital rectal examination during the year of the study. With wider application, a reduction in mortality might well emerge.

526. Lehrer S. Clinical trial of rectal self-examination. *Arch Intern Med.* 1979;139:1194.

In view of the above (*see* reference 525), no more than one per one billion examinations can prove to be lifesaving. The procedure defies human aesthetic and athletic norms, not just the agility of elderly persons, as the author recognizes.

527. Rosen L. Physical examination of the anorectum: a systematic technique. *Dis Colon Rectum.* 1990;33:439-40.

Not new information but a useful synthesis.

528. Schneiderman H. Basal cell carcinoma of the anus, and aspects of anorectal examination. *Consultant.* 1996;36:2007-13.

Emphasizes a modality as underused for the anorectal examination as for the abdominal examination.

529. Stearns MW. Digital rectal examination. *CA Cancer J Clin.* 1974;24:100-3.

Housestaff who record only "rectal: guaiac negative" could learn to extract 50 times as much information by studying this article.

530. Wilt TJ, Cutler AF. Physician performance and patient perceptions during the rectal examination. *J Gen Intern Med.* 1991;6:514-7.

Resident physicians in a good program know little to nothing about why to do this examination or how to do it comfortably. The need for educational measures is glaring.

Fecal occult-blood testing

531. Anonymous. Screening for colorectal cancer—United States, 1992–1993, and new guidelines. *MMWR*. 1996;45:107-10 (reprinted in *JAMA*. 1996; 275:830-1).

Gives data showing that only a fraction of at-risk adults have had fecal occult blood testing, digital rectal examination, or proctoscopy according to self-report by a massive telephone survey. There is a clear need to increase these measures. The lack of consensus that rectal examination has a real role to play is striking.

532. Kulbaski MJ, Goold SD, Tecce MA, et al. Oral iron and the Hemoccult test: a controversy on the teaching wards [Letter]. *N Engl J Med*. 1989; 320:1500.

Discusses how in normal housestaff and medical students, standard oral ferrous sulfate did not produce positive Hemoccult tests, although a suspension of the tablets did so when applied directly—not via the intestines of the study participants—to the reagent card.

533. McDonnell M, Elta G. More on oral iron and the hemoccult test [Letter]. *N Engl J Med*. 1989;321:1684.

A short follow-up that invokes the difference between soluble and insoluble salts of varying valence to account for the in vivo failure to replicate the in vitro reaction. Dilution of the iron would also make sense.

534. Longstreth GF. Checking for "the occult" with a finger: a procedure of little value. *J Clin Gastroenterol*. 1988;10:133-4.

Discusses how occult blood tests on grossly normal-appearing feces may have unacceptably high rates of false-positive and false-negative results. The gross appearance of the stool needs to be recorded in patients with gastrointestinal bleeding because it provides a datum separate from occult blood testing.

535. Selby JV, Friedman GD, Quesenberry CP Jr, Weiss NS. Effect of fecal occult blood testing on mortality from colorectal cancer: a case-control study. *Ann Intern Med*. 1993;118:1-6.

This study of patients with fatal colorectal cancer and age-matched controls gives wide confidence intervals and therefore is a bit cautious in recommending expanding the role of this test in screening. Most clinicians would find it intolerable to omit testing stool recovered on the examining glove after rectal examination done for any indication including screening, at least yearly in persons older than 50 years.

536. Winawer SJ. Colorectal cancer screening comes of age [Editorial]. *N Engl J Med.* **1993;328:1416-7.**

At long last, there is a study showing unequivocally reduced mortality from colon cancer in persons who have had annual fecal occult blood tests compared with those who have not.

Examination of the prostate per rectum

537. Clements R, Griffiths GJ, Peeling WB, et al. How accurate is the index finger? A comparison of digital and ultrasound examination of the prostatic nodule. *Clin Radiol.* **1988;39:87-9.**

Describes how sensitivity in separating benign from malignant nodules is identical for these two kinds of examinations. This contradicts the conventional wisdom that more cancers are detected by imaging than by palpation, perhaps because of characteristics of the patient group studied: The patients studied were those with a palpable nodule. *Specificity* in this group is greater when ultrasonography is used. Surprisingly, intraprostatic calcium does not produce false-positive digital rectal examinations for cancer.

538. Crawford ED, Schutz MJ, Clejan S, et al. The effect of digital rectal examination on prostate-specific antigen levels. *JAMA.* **1992;267:2227-8.**

Discusses how the effect of the digital rectal examination on prostate-specific antigen levels is not clinically significant: Only in those persons who already have high basal levels that would call for investigation does the level increase with this examination. Sometimes the level *falls* (!) after examination. Results cannot be extrapolated to postmassage or postcystoscopy levels. The number of other papers on this topic is staggering.

539. Friedman GD, Hiatt RA, Quesenberry CP Jr, Selby JV. Case-control study of screening for prostatic cancer by digital rectal examinations. *Lancet.* **1991;337:1526-9.**

A look at the interval between prostatic palpation testing in patients presenting with low stages of prostate cancer as compared to patients presenting with high stages of prostate cancer. More frequent rectal examinations seem not to preclude presentation with established metastatic disease.

540. Sutton MA, Gibbons RP, Correa RJ. Is deleting the digital rectal examination a good idea? *West J Med.* 1991;155:43-6.

Provides some evidence that prostate cancer may be more often curable if discovered by physical examination rather than after the development of sentinel symptoms, which all too often arise only from osseous metastases. Contradicts conclusions of reference 539.

541. Guinan P, Bush I, Ray V, et al. The accuracy of the rectal examination in the diagnosis of prostate carcinoma. *N Engl J Med*. 1980;303:499-503.

Describes how in a defined population, rectal examination outdistanced other tests in separating cancer from benign hyperplasia.

542. Mueller EJ, Crain TW, Thompson IM, Rodriguez FR. An evaluation of serial digital rectal examinations in screening for prostate cancer. *J Urol*. 1988;140:1445-7.

An ill-conducted study attempts to give scientific credibility to the common wisdom that new cancers found 1 year after a last negative digital rectal examination are more frequently curable than those found after a longer interval.

543. Smith DS, Catalona WJ. Interexaminer variability of digital rectal examination in detecting prostate cancer. *Urology*. 1995;45:70-4.

Describes discordance between back-to-back blinded examinations by two urologists, especially if one or both are in residency. Several subsequently biopsy-proven cancers were suspected by only one of the two examiners, and a biopsy would not otherwise have been done because the prostate-specific antigen was low. No mention of whether palpable abnormality correlated with positive biopsy: patients had four-quadrant biopsies each.

Male Genitals

Hernia

544. Rourke JT. The laughing hernia sign. *Can Med Assoc J.* **1988;138:721.**

A delightful discovery, exemplary of the opportunities to enhance the repertoire of signs simply by attentive observation, even in the jaded world of the 1990s!

Penis

545. Ackerman AB, Kornberg R. Pearly penile papules: acral angiofibromas. *Arch Dermatol.* **1973;108:673-5.**

Discusses tiny, raised dots arranged circumferentially around the corona. Innocuous but need to be recognized to avoid futile searches for sexually transmitted disease where it is not present.

546. Schneiderman H. Pearly penile papules. *Consultant.* 1991;31(7):39-40.

A little ring of harmless nubbins liable to misinterpretation as signs of venereal disease or infection.

547. Barrasso R, De Brux J, Croissant O, Orth G. High prevalence of papillomavirus-associated penile intraepithelial neoplasia in sexual partners of women with cervical intraepithelial neoplasia. *N Engl J Med.* **1987; 317:916-23.**

Well-illustrated discussion. The oncogenic papillomaviruses have changed the risk profile for penile cancer as well as for cervical and vulvar carcinoma.

548. Horan DB, Redman JF, Jansen GT. Papulosquamous lesions of glans penis. *Urology.* **1984;23:1-4.**

Discusses how a scaly plaque on the glans may be a harbinger of a systemic dermatosis and warrants evaluation of the remaining skin, the nails, and the oral mucosa as much as it warrants consideration of possible venereal disease. Includes several useful illustrations.

549. **Ratzan RM, Donaldson MC, Foster JH, Walzak MP. The blue scrotum sign of Bryant: a diagnostic clue to ruptured abdominal aortic aneurysm.** *J Emerg Med.* **1987;5:323-9.**

Describes how extravasation of blood in the retroperitoneum may lead to nontraumatic discoloration beneath intact penile or scrotal epithelium.

550. **Rosemberg SK. Subclinical papilloma viral infection of male genitalia.** *Urology.* **1985;26:554-7.**

Discusses how a disclosing solution of 5% acetic acid will produce characteristic whitening in areas of flat condyloma that could not be recognized otherwise. Some other conditions and topical applications produce false-positive tests.

Prostate (see Rectum)

Testes, adnexae, vas, scrotum

551. **Amelar RD, Dubin L. Importance of careful palpation of vas deferens [Letter].** *Urology.* **1974;4:495.**

Significant findings regard fertility and systemic illness or health, as well as purely local problems. Absent or malformed vasa, for example, are seen in virtually all cases of cystic fibrosis.

552. Donohue RE, Fauver HE. Unilateral absence of the vas deferens: a useful clinical sign. *JAMA.* 1989;261:1180-2.

The association with ipsilateral renal agenesis is quite striking. Complementary to the search for bilateral vas pathology.

553. **Benson RC Jr, Tomera KM. Significance of testicular size.** *Med Aspects Human Sexuality.* **1985;19:165-74.**

Listing and some discussion of causes of small as well as oversized testes, beyond the cryptorchidism and tumor that first come to mind for internists. Includes some material on testicular texture as an aid to this assessment.

554. **Najmaldin A, Burge DM. Acute idiopathic scrotal oedema: incidence, manifestations and aetiology.** *Br J Surg.* **1987;74:634-5.**

Describes this little-known condition that has a characteristic bright pink color, principally found in prepubertal boys.

555. Rosemberg SK. Sexually transmitted papillomaviral infections: IV. The white scrotum. *Urology.* 1989;33:462-4.

Observations that parallel observations made on the penis (*see* reference 550).

556. Roy CR II, Wilson T, Raife M, Horne D. Varicocele as the presenting sign of an abdominal mass. *J Urol.* 1989;141:597-9.

The pathophysiology that produces this sign is compression of the testicular vein. The sign is an old one for (late-stage) renal cell carcinoma. Some authors consider right-sided varicoceles more important, others, left-sided varicoceles.

557. Wheeler RA, Atwell JD. Horizontal testis with a varicocele: a new physical sign. *Br J Surg.* 1991;78:225.

Discusses how a dozen boys with varicocele had the ipsilateral testis lying horizontally and the contralateral testis in the normal vertical alignment. The mechanism of relationship is speculative, and the separate significance, if any, is unknown.

558. Zornow DH, Landes RR. Scrotal palpation. *Am Fam Physician.* 1981; 23:150-4.

Includes material on inspection and transillumination as well as on palpation. Also discusses techniques, characteristic findings, and differential points.

Pelvic Examination and Gynecologic Evaluation

General material: uterine and cervical examination

559. Broadmore J, Carr-Gregg M, Hutton JD. Vaginal examinations: women's experiences and preferences. *N Z Med J*. 1986;99:8-10.

A survey (again) documents what patients appreciate—namely, empathy and explanation—and what they dislike. Some surprises, including that most patients preferred not to have a third person (chaperone) present, and that the frequency of this preference was not significantly correlated with the sex of the examiner.

560. Deneke M, Wheeler L, Wagner G, et al. An approach to relearning the pelvic examination. *J Fam Pract*. 1982;14:782-3.

Trained patient-instructors offer unique insights on both technique and interpersonal manner. This article concerns updating practitioners' skills. Similar approaches succeed with students and with internal medicine residents.

561. Levitt MA. An evaluation of clinical variables in determining the need for pelvic examination in the emergency department. *Ann Emerg Med*. 1991;20:351-4.

Discusses how in a group of some 250 women visiting an urban emergency department with abdominal pain, the presence of left lower quadrant pain or tenderness was associated with increased risk of pelvic disease, as was any history of vaginal discharge, dysmenorrhea, or menorrhagia. By contrast, the presence of right upper quadrant tenderness was associated with reduced relative risk. However, this should not lead to any change in clinician behavior: omitting the pelvic examination in any woman with abdominal pain still would not make good sense.

562. Magee J. The pelvic examination: a view from the other end of the table. *Ann Intern Med*. 1975;83:563-4.

Angry, well-reasoned, and crucial insights on the failure to afford dignity to patients. Specific recommendations.

563. **Meeks GR, Cesare CD, Bates GW. Palpable uterine artery pulsation as a clinical indicator of early pregnancy.** *J Reproduc Med.* **1995;40:194-6.**

Discusses how, while one is performing bimanual palpation, the second and third digits, in the lateral vaginal fornices, may seek pulsations palpable with minimal pressure on the parametrium. The predictive value of a positive examination is not clinically definitive, whereas women want 100% certainty. The study is well conducted, the outlook sound, and the historical review of other physical signs of early pregnancy is the best available.

564. **Newman L. Pelvic exam: Technical aspects and doctor–patient interaction. Farmington, CT: Biomedical Communications, University of Connecticut School of Medicine, 1989 (WP 141L 438 VHS library call number).**

Meticulously detailed description of the practical and pragmatic as well as the psychological necessities for deriving valid information. Helps one make the procedure as little unpleasant as possible for the patient. Worthwhile for close review by even the most experienced practitioner.

565. **Nolting WE, Moodley J, Gouws E. Naked eye screening for cervical intra-epithelial abnormalities: a preliminary report.** *Trop Doct.* **1995; 25(3):130-1.**

Discusses an exciting idea that has not yet reached fruition: to make the best use of scarce Papanicolaou smears in developing countries by selecting which women need them using (unspecified) criteria on inspection per speculum. Although all the in situ cancers were predicted correctly, the predictive value of a positive test was very poor, and the sensitivity for human papillomavirus infection was low. Further work involving pretreatment with acetic acid may yield more applicable results.

566. **Peipert JF. Pap smears: whom you should screen, and how to do it better.** *Consultant.* **1994;34:717-24.**

Briefly addresses the benefits, problems, and technique of Pap smears. Tabulates Bethesda classification system of cytologic specimens, grading of cervical epithelial neoplasia, and human papillomavirus types carrying various oncogenic risks.

567. **Primrose RB. Taking the tension out of pelvic exams.** *Am J Nurs.* **1984;84(1):72-4.**

Among the best suggestions here: that the instruction to relax is almost useless; that covers on the stirrups make for comfort, as do posters and other nonmedical decorations; that a running commentary is usually appreciated; that palpation of the cervix beforehand assists comfortable and accurate speculum placement (however, use water as lubricant, because jellies ruin the cytology specimen); that Scopettes Junior applicators help clean out copious discharge to help one to see underlying tissue; and that the patient needs to be reminded to slide her hips and bottom backward after the examination and before sitting up.

568. **Sanders RM, Nakajima ST. An unusual late presentation of imperforate hymen.** *Obstet Gynecol.* **1994;83:896-8.**

Discusses how erroneous ultrasound imaging misled the gynecologist. The patient had become able to have intercourse after vaginal dilation. Definitive diagnosis and management awaited a second, perceptive physical examination.

569. **Sargent E. Unusual pelvic pain apparently cured by pelvic examination [Letter].** *West J Med.* **1980;133:80.**

A therapeutic effect not mediated by achieving diagnosis or by allaying fear.

570. Schneiderman H. Pelvic pain cured by pelvic examination [Letter]. *West J Med.* 1984;141:686.

Follow-up letter proposes that rupture of paratubal cysts may be responsible for the cessation of pain.

571. **Sturman MF. Pelvic examination versus fiberoptic laparoscopy: a fictional study of patient preference in 1534 women.** *J Clin Gastroenterol.* **1988;10:612-3.**

One of the few humorous approaches to the issues of physical examination and technology.

572. **Wallis LA, Jacobson JS. The hundred years are up.** *J Am Med Wom Assoc.* **1984;39:59, 62.**

Discusses the timeliness of several issues relating to women's health and women physicians, including pelvic examination.

History

573. **Ramoska EA, Sacchetti AD, Nepp M. Reliability of patient history in determining the possibility of pregnancy.** *Ann Emerg Med.* **1989;18:48-50.**

In the population studied, positive beta-human chorionic gonadotropin (beta-HCG) tests were found in every tenth woman who affirmed that she could not possibly be pregnant! Probably applies to a lesser (but still considerable) extent to unselected populations.

Positioning

574. Drife JO. Lateral thinking in gynaecology. *Br Med J.* **1988;296:807-8.**

Part of the debate about supine versus left lateral positioning.

575. Swartz WH. The semi-sitting position for pelvic examination [Letter]. *JAMA.* **1984;251:1163.**

Addresses its issue with clear, nonpolemical thought: the patient can make better eye contact when in the semi-sitting position. The examining table sometimes cannot accommodate this need.

External pelvic examination (vulvar examination)

576. Pincus SH. Vulvar dermatoses and pruritus vulvae. *Dermatol Clin.* **1992; 10:297-308.**

Covers less material on the vulvar dystrophies than some readers might want. Good discussion of an often confusing chief complaint and a close review of skin lesions in the area, complementary to the author's encyclopedic chapter in the textbook of dermatology in general medicine edited by Fitzpatrick (reference 160).

577. Turner MLC. Vulvar manifestations of systemic diseases. *Dermatol Clin.* **1992;10:445-58.**

Part of what can be learned from pelvic examination, even of the woman unable to assume the lithotomy position. Well illustrated and well proportioned catalogue of infections, immune disorders, endocrinopathies including estrogen deprivation, and nonsquamous neoplasms that can have vulvar signs. Every bit as useful to the nongynecologist and the nondermatologist as it is to gynecologists and dermatologists.

Adnexal examination and findings

578. Barber HR. The postmenopausal palpable ovary syndrome. *Compr Ther.* **1979;5:58-60.**

Argues that a palpable "normal-sized" ovary 3 years after the onset of menopause requires exclusion of cancer. Today, ultrasonography makes laparotomy for this consideration unnecessary, but the need to investigate persists.

579. Tyden G, Groth CG. **Pancreatic graft failure due to pelvic examination [Letter].** *Lancet.* **1987;1:812.**

Describes the way in which awareness of use of the iliac fossa for various heterotopic grafts can prevent this complication.

Chaperones

580. Palmer RN. **The need for chaperones: is greatest during intimate examination [Letter].** *BMJ.* **1993;307:1353.**

The roles of patient ignorance (when a body part remote from chief complaint is legitimately examined), of innuendo, and of comments in leading to unfounded complaints of indecency.

581. Simmons P. The need for chaperones: doctors need protection from assault [Letter]. *BMJ.* 1993;307:1353.

Police as well as staff can help as two-way protective chaperones when there is fear that the *physician* may become the object of the assault.

582. Cole FH. The need for chaperones: chaperones are expensive and time consuming [Letter]. *BMJ.* 1993;307:1353.

Curmudgeonly rejoinder.

583. Protheroe D. The need for chaperones: chaperones valuable in difficult psychiatric interviews [Letter]. *BMJ.* 1993;307:1353.

Only the British could phrase it so well: "A stoical chaperone of the same sex as the patient may be invaluable in separating an ill patient from an embarrassed male or female doctor."

Urinary incontinence evaluation (both sexes)

584. Bergman A, Bader K. **Reliability of the patient's history in the diagnosis of urinary incontinence.** *Int J Gynaecol Obstet.* **1990;32:255-9.**

A long questionnaire is compared with formal urodynamic testing. Symptoms and factors are identified that can misleadingly mimic stress incontinence and detrusor instability. Shows that the history, taken in isolation, can misdirect evaluation.

585. Dawson C, Whitfield H. **Urological evaluation. (ABC of Urology.)** *BMJ.* **1996;312:695-8.**

Material on symptoms is particularly useful in providing concise definitions and inferences. Defines strangury (recurrent painful desire to void with only a small volume passed each time) and pis-en-deux, the desire to void again shortly after doing so, typically a symptom of high post-void residual bladder urine volume.

586. DuBeau CE, Resnick NM. Evaluation of the causes and severity of geriatric incontinence: a critical appraisal. *Urol Clin North Am.* **1991; 18:243-56.**

Focuses on the whole issue of work-up. Many comments are so brief as to exclude the newcomer to the field. Material on the limits and uses of the history and physical examination is quite useful.

Locomotor System and Limbs

General

587. Ad Hoc Committee. Guidelines for the initial evaluation of the adult patient with acute musculoskeletal symptoms. *Arthritis Rheum.* 1996;39:1-8.

Focuses more on history than on physical examination, and more on laboratory than on either. Valuable, among many other reasons, for reminding one that the combination of point tenderness, reduced active range of motion, and preserved passive range of motion suggests bursitis, tendinitis, or muscle injury.

588. Gomez JE, Landry GL, Bernhardt DT. Critical evaluation of the 2-minute orthopedic screening examination. *AJDC.* 1993;147:1109-13.

Discusses how in employing a very brief method to detect latent injuries that might preclude participation in sports in collegiate athletes, clinicians missed many important lesions and overdiagnosed several shoulder asymmetries as disease. The history proved more potent than physical examination.

589. Greidinger EL, Hellmann DB. Arthritis: what to emphasize on the rheumatologic exam. *Consultant.* 1995;35:1609-17.

A few striking photographs and some help in distinguishing osteoarthrosis from gout, among other issues. Makes as much use of history as of physical examination, the title notwithstanding. No substitute for a textbook of musculoskeletal examination.

590. Hoppenfeld S. *Physical Examination of the Spine and Extremities.* **Norwalk, CT: Appleton-Century-Crofts, 1976.**

The reference text on the orthopedic examination. Crisp, well focused, and well illustrated.

591. Mollan RAB, McCullagh GC, Wilson RI. A critical appraisal of auscultation of human joints. *Clin Orthop.* 1982;170:231-7.

Fascinating review of the application of the stethoscope to the detection of articular pathology over the past century and more. Investigates the barriers, which are not just skin friction noise and ambient noise, but intrinsic frequency of the sounds produced, in a range better appreciated by the vibratory sensors of the fingers than by either ear, stethoscope, or microphone.

592. **Polley HF, Hunder GG.** *Rheumatologic Interviewing and Physical Examination of the Joints.* **2nd ed. Philadelphia: WB Saunders; 1978.**

Exhaustive compendium. Reference work for any particular site or sign.

593. **Shapiro MS, Trebich C, Shilo L, Shenkman L. Myalgias and muscle contractures as the presenting signs of Addison's disease.** *Postgrad Med J.* **1988;64:222-3.**

Discusses a little-appreciated aspect. Restates the need to consider hypoadrenalism, even with normal electrolyte values.

Back

594. **Blower PW, Griffin AJ. Clinical sacroiliac tests in ankylosing spondylitis and other causes of low back pain—2 studies.** *Ann Rheum Dis.* **1984;43:192-5.**

Describes how four signs were tested in attempting to distinguish ankylosing spondylitis from more conventional low back pain. Tenderness to pressure over the anterior superior iliac spines and over the lower sacrum supported ankylosing spondylitis.

595. **Dyck P, Doyle JB Jr. "Bicycle test" of van Gelderen in diagnosis of intermittent cauda equina compression syndrome.** *J Neurosurg.* **1977;46:667-70.**

Seeking to distinguish positional pseudoclaudication of cauda equina compression from conventional arterial insufficiency pain, the author asked a man who experienced pain on walking to achieve comparable exercise on a stationary bicycle. Leaning backward, the patient was in agony; hunching forward over the handlebars, he had no pain. Includes dramatic photographs of relief of myelographic blockage by flexion of the spine.

596. **Katz JN, Dalgas M, Stucki G, et al. Degenerative lumbar spinal stenosis: diagnostic value of the history and physical examination.** *Arthritis Rheum.* **1995;38:1236-41.**

Demonstrates that older age, severe lower-limb pain, precipitation of pain by 30 seconds of lumbar extension, and relief of pain when seated increased the likelihood ratio of spinal stenosis. Wide-based gait and abnormal Romberg test were also suggestive of the diagnosis. The study population was composed of referral patients with a very high prevalence of imaging-established spinal stenosis, so the results may not be generalizable.

597. McCombe PF, Fairbank JCT, Cockersole BC, Pynsent PB. Reproducibility of physical signs in low-back pain. *Spine.* **1989;14:908–18.**

When comparing the findings of two orthopedic surgeons with each other, or of one with a physiotherapist, best agreement was achieved in the cases of lordosis, pain on flexion and lateral bending, and straight-leg-raising tests. Root tension signs were less reproducible, as was soft-tissue tenderness.

598. Murtagh J. Physical signs in low back pain [Pictorial essay]. *Aust Fam Physician.* **1989;18:1561-2.**

A small catalogue of what inspection and palpation can reveal, including lateral deviation of the back, fixed flexion, scoliosis, muscle spasm, a step in the spine in spondylolisthesis, and special signs for nonorganic origin. Unfortunately, most patients lack any of these helpful signs.

599. Simkin PA. Simian stance: a sign of spinal stenosis. *Lancet.* **1982;2:652-3.**

Discusses how flexion of hips, knees, and lower back sometimes relieves pressure on nerve roots. Because lumbar spinal stenosis can be difficult to diagnose when there are no neurologic deficits, this posture can help. Flexion of the neck is a usual concomitant, and neck extension as well as back extension can worsen symptoms. The patient may voluntarily straighten up for a short period, so one must look for ability to sustain rather than simply to attain the upright posture.

600. Van den Hoogen HMM, Koes BW, Van Eijk JTM, Bouter LM. On the accuracy of history, physical examination, and erythrocyte sedimentation rate in diagnosing low back pain in general practice: a criteria-based review of the literature. *Spine.* **1995;20:318-27.**

Shows that individual signs and symptoms do not help much in identifying the small subset of patients with low back pain that has nonmechanical causes, such as ankylosing spondylitis, metastatic disease, or radiculopathy. Further studies are needed.

601. Waddell G, McCulloch JA, Kummel E, Venner RM. Nonorganic physical signs in low-back pain. *Spine.* **1980;5:117-25.**

Although personality test results of the patients studied suggested dysfunction, the authors did not establish whether organic back disease coexisted and explained their positive "nonorganic" back findings, nor did they describe what kind of follow-up might have clarified residual concerns.

Lower limbs

General

602. Olofinboba KA, Schneiderman H. Elephantiasis nostras. *Consultant.* 1995;35:1015-9.

Discussion of this highly disfiguring but treatment-amenable variant of hyperkeratosis and ichthyosis due to chronic venous or lymphatic congestion or both.

603. Witte MH, Witte CL. Massive obesity simulating lymphedema. *N Engl J Med* [Images in Clinical Medicine]. 1992;327:1927.

Pictorial presentation of a case resolved by radionuclide lymphangiography and magnetic resonance imaging of the lower extremities. See also combined review in reference 604.

604. Loughlin V. Massive obesity simulating lymphedema [Letter]. *N Engl J Med.* 1993;328:1496.

This letter improves the differentiation between lymphedema and lipedema (a misnomer).

605. Reilly DT, Wolfe JHN. The swollen leg. *BMJ.* 1991;303:1462-5.

Although this "ABC of Vascular Diseases" mini-review covers a wide range, it focuses chiefly on the chronically swollen leg and the clinical features of lymphedema versus those of the postphlebitic leg and other venous disorders.

Hip

606. Murtagh J. Diagnosis of early osteoarthritis of hip joint: the four-step stress test. *Aust Fam Physician.* 1990;19:389.

States that internal rotation, abduction, and extension are usually the first three of the six cardinal motions of the joint to become symptomatic, and advocates a four-step test. This article is weakened by an apparent typographic error: the word *prone* appears where context and photograph suggest that *supine* is meant.

607. Peltier LF. The diagnosis of fractures of the hip and femur by auscultatory percussion. *Clin Orthop.* 1977;123:9-11.

Discusses an effective method, consisting of ausculting at the symphysis pubis while lightly tapping each patella in turn with one finger. Markedly reduced sound transmission supports the impression of ipsilateral fracture. This method is most helpful if radiography is not easily available or is indeterminate. False-positive results from prosthetic hips, which the author did not discuss in this article published 20 years ago, are now common and must be kept in mind.

Knees

608. Ike RW, O'Rourke KS. Compartment-directed physical examination of the knee can predict articular cartilage abnormalities disclosed by needle arthroscopy. *Arthritis Rheum.* **1995;38:917-25.**

Describes how if the examiner can feel the crepitus while holding the distal tibia, bone-on-bone grating will occur, something of some therapeutic and prognostic import. Expertise in the maneuvers described in this article may be sustained only by specialists in musculoskeletal medicine and surgery.

609. Lonergan RP. Tips of the trade: detecting patellar surface irregularities. *Ortho Rev.* 1992;21:253-4.

Discusses how recognition of patellar alterations signifying chondromalacia can be enhanced by making a little megaphone of a cupped hand, which amplifies and transmits crepitus with movement. It is not clear whether this is useful for the generalist.

610. Mann G, Finsterbush A, Frankl U, et al. A method of diagnosing small amounts of fluid in the knee. *J Bone Joint Surg Br.* **1991;73-B:346-7.**

Carefully stated and illustrated; perhaps an advance over the older, well-known bulge test described in reference 590.

611. Rothenberg MH, Graf BK. Evaluation of acute knee injuries. *Postgrad Med.* **1993;93:75-86.**

Describes in considerable detail physical examination techniques and findings as they pertain to the acutely injured knee. Graphs on anatomy enliven this useful presentation.

Ankle, shin, calf

612. Brady HR, Quigley C, Stafford FJ, et al. Popliteal cyst rupture and the pseudothrombophlebitis syndrome. *Ann Emerg Med.* **1987;16:1151-4.**

Discusses how popliteal cyst rupture and deep venous thrombosis of the calf are sometimes clinically indistinguishable. States that a popliteal mass or a perimalleolar crescentic ecchymosis, highly suggestive of ruptured Baker's cyst (*see* reference 614), is all too seldom observed. A history of arthritis of the ipsilateral knee may be a helpful clue, but differentiation still relies on imaging technology.

613. Frost HM, Hanson CA. Technique for testing the drawer sign in the ankle. *Clin Orthop.* **1977;123:49-51.**

For effective performance of ankle drawer tests, it is mandatory that all muscles acting on the ankle be fully relaxed. Useful explanatory photographs are presented.

614. **Good AE, Pozderac RV. Ecchymosis of the lower leg: a sign of hemarthrosis with synovial rupture.** *Arthritis Rheum.* **1977;20:1009-13.**

Describes the crescent sign, produced by fascial restraint of gravitationally settling hemorrhagic synovial fluid extravasated from a ruptured Baker's cyst. The sign can be seen about either the lateral or the medial malleolus.

615. **Henry JA, Altmann P. Assessment of hypoproteinaemic oedema: a simple physical sign.** *Br Med J.* **1978;1:890-2.**

This study, using a cleverly conceived device, shows that faster pitting and faster recovery characterize hypoproteinemic edema compared with edema caused by elevated venous pressure.

616. **Humbert P, Dupond JL, Carbillet JP. Pretibial myxedema: an overlapping clinical manifestation of autoimmune thyroid disease.** *Am J Med.* **1987;83:1170-1.**

This feature is now recognized in a few cases of Hashimoto thyroiditis as well as in the more familiar setting of Graves' disease.

617. **Ninia JG, Goldberg TL. Assessing varicose and telangiectatic leg veins.** *IM (Internal Medicine for the Specialist).* **1996;17:15-6, 23.**

Short review on the bedside evaluation of varicose veins.

Feet and toes

618. **Brown C. A review of subcalcaneal heel pain and plantar fasciitis.** *Austr Fam Physician.* **1996;25:875-85.**

Discussion of the competing diagnoses, with reference to anatomic diagrams. Reference 626 is also illuminating.

619. **Caputo GM, Cavanagh PR, Ulbrecht JS, et al. Assessment and management of foot disease in patients with diabetes.** *N Engl J Med.* **1994; 331:854-60.**

In addition to being an exceptionally lucid and insightful review of its topic, this paper describes the monofilament test for loss of protective sensation and alludes to the test of probing for bone described in reference 620.

620. **Grayson ML, Gibbons GW, Balogh K, et al. Probing to bone in infected pedal ulcers: a clinical sign of underlying osteomyelitis in diabetic patients.** *JAMA.* **1995;273:721-3.**

Because visible bone in the base of a diabetic foot ulcer is insensitive albeit specific for osteomyelitis, the authors palpated with an eyed probe to enhance yield and found that probe-palpable bone in the base confers a high enough probability to justify antibiotic treatment for this condition without requiring imaging studies.

621. **Johnson FL. The painful foot: an overview of podalgia.** *Aust Fam Physician.* **1987;16:1083-8.**

Differential diagnosis of podalgia, with several suggestions to improve the yield of history, examination, and investigations.

622. **Kurzrock R, Cohen PR. Erythromelalgia: review of clinical characteristics and pathophysiology.** *Am J Med.* **1991;91:416-22.**

Describes erythromelalgia as burning, warmth, and redness usually of the feet, although the condition can also occur elsewhere in the body. In adults, 40% of patients with this condition have underlying myeloproliferative disorders. Mysteriously, the erythromelalgia can precede the development of thrombocytosis.

623. **Mahowald ML. Examination of the foot in rheumatic disease.** *Postgrad Med.* **1986;79:258-61, 264.**

Anatomic review, with description of examination techniques and injection sites.

624. **O'Keeffe ST, Woods B O'B, Breslin DJ, Tsapatsaris NP. Blue toe syndrome: causes and management.** *Arch Intern Med.* **1992;152:2197-202.**

Although slightly redundant, this is the best available review on the "blue toes" of atheroembolism.

625. Scher RK. Jogger's toe. *Int J Dermatol.* 1978;17:719-20.

Describes yet another ecchymosis to be recognized, and not to be confused with blue toe syndrome.

626. **Zatouroff M, Bouffler LE.** *A Colour Atlas of the Foot in Clinical Diagnosis.* **London: Wolfe Publishing; 1992.**

A fruitful collaboration of an internist and a podiatrist to show an immense array of foot conditions, with mention of the systemic significance of some.

Upper limbs

627. **Alpert JS, Krous HF, Dalen JE, et al. Pathogenesis of Osler's nodes.** *Ann Intern Med.* **1976;85:471-3.**

Comments on clinical recognition. Makes the case that Osler nodes arise from embolism of infective vegetations, rather than immunologically.

628. Durkan JA. A new diagnostic test for carpal tunnel syndrome. *J Bone Joint Surg Am.* **1991;73(A):535-8.**

The test described in this article is accomplished by sustained pressure applied (usually) by both of the examiner's thumbs to the flexor retinaculum. In this analysis, both sensitivity and specificity exceeded the discredited Tinel sign and the more respectable Phalen sign. Enthusiastic presentation includes speculating that the "false-positives" with the sign may be true-positives with false-negative electrophysiologic tests. Clearly requires replication and evaluation by others.

629. Elliott BG. Finkelstein's test: a descriptive error that can produce a false-positive. *J Hand Surg Br.* **1992;17:481-2.**

Discusses how with this test, the examiner should grip the patient's thumb and quickly abduct the hand ulnarward, producing excruciating pain over the styloid tip of the radius. The movement with thumb folded into the hand was devised to produce pain in normal hosts; excess vigor in the correct version may also produce false-positives.

630. Murtagh J. De Quervain's tenosynovitis and Finkelstein's test. *Aust Fam Physician.* 1989;18:1552.

One of many published articles that misstate the test method.

631. Farrior JB III, Silverman ME. A consideration of the differences between a Janeway's lesion and an Osler's node in infectious endocarditis. *Chest.* **1976;70:239-43.**

Clarifies these vanishing signs.

632. Yee J, McAllister K. The utility of Osler's nodes in the diagnosis of infective endocarditis. *Chest.* 1987;92:751-2.

Discusses how Osler nodes help make the diagnosis, even when "the echo is negative." They can be cultured to find the organism, sometimes successfully despite negative blood cultures.

633. Foley AE. Tennis elbow. *Am Fam Physician.* **1993;48:281-8.**

Includes descriptions of several useful signs, such as the "coffee cup sign" and the use of carrying a heavy book to induce pain; fails to cite the Coen sign by name.

634. Katz GA, Peter JB, Pearson CM, Adams WS. The shoulder-pad sign: a diagnostic feature of amyloid arthropathy. *N Engl J Med.* **1973; 288:354-5.**

No new information has emerged since these two case reports were published more than 20 years ago.

635. Katz JN, Larson MG, Sabra A, et al. The carpal tunnel syndrome: diagnostic utility of the history and physical examination findings. *Ann Intern Med.* 1990;112:321-7.

As most of us have noticed from clinical experience, no single component of the history or examination definitively "clinches" the diagnosis of carpal tunnel syndrome. In this study, conducted at a referral neurophysiology laboratory, the operational characteristics of symptoms and signs were of limited utility; a combination of tests should be used. The diagnostic impression of experienced clinicians remains invaluable, and neurophysiologic studies continue to be an important resource for clinicians.

636. Latimer HA, Taft TN. Shoulder disorders: six questions and a hands-on examination are keys to diagnosis. *Consultant.* 1994;34:1305-16.

Simple review with practical tips on the physical examination. The "six shoulder questions" relate to the disorder and its onset, its patterns of recurrence, its relationship to trauma, diurnal fluctuations in symptoms, aggravating factors, and degree of engendered disability.

637. Shmerling RH, Stern SH, Gravallese EM, Kantrowitz FG. Tophaceous deposition in the finger pads without gouty arthritis. *Arch Intern Med.* 1988;148:1830-2.

Case reports of four elderly women without joint involvement. Definitions of prevalence, mechanisms, and predictive values await further studies and will determine when the sign is worth seeking.

638. Silverman ME, Hurst JW. The hand and the heart. *Am J Cardiol.* 1968;22:718-28.

Extraordinarily wide-ranging consideration. The so-called update in the textbook is now sadly reduced to scattered parts in the chapter by O'Rourke RA, Silverman ME, and Schlant RC, "General Examination of the Patient," chapter 10 in the text edited by Schlant RC and Alexander RW, *Hurst's The Heart, Arteries and Veins.* 8th ed. New York: McGraw-Hill; 1994.

Neurologic Examination

General material and textbooks

639. Chimowitz MI, Logigian EL, Caplan LR. The accuracy of bedside neurological diagnoses. *Ann Neurol.* 1990;28:78-85.

Provocative, probing, and intriguing study. Unfortunately, the results may be a bit intimidating to non-neurologists. Some general principles emerge.

640. Chynn EW, Kao K-P, Liu R-S. Hepatitis B transmission by neurologic pin testing [Letter]. *Neurology.* 1993;43:1618.

The first scientific proof of the recoverability of the agent from a neurologic examining instrument; supports what has been asserted earlier on the basis of common sense.

641. Chan AW, MacFarlane IA, Bowsher D, Campbell JA. Weighted needle pinprick sensory thresholds: a simple test of sensory function in diabetic peripheral neuropathy. *J Neurol Neurosurg Psychiatry.* 1992;55:56-9.

The authors' insights on this test are worthwhile, but the problem with the test is that it is subject to sloppy performance: if the needles are not replaced as the authors advocate, perhaps because the practice is busy—which is just the setting in which they advocate doing this test—disease transmission could occur, as per reference 640 and the many cautions about HIV.

642. DeMyer W. *Technique of the Neurologic Examination: A Programmed Text.* 4th ed. New York: McGraw-Hill, Inc.; 1994.

Quirky, original, creative, and user-friendly. Best used in tandem with Haerer's book (reference 645) rather than as an alternative to it.

643. Goldstein LB, Matchar DB. Clinical assessment of stroke. (The Rational Clinical Examination.) *JAMA.* 1994;271:1114-20.

An interesting review of the precision and accuracy of the clinical examination in the evaluation of stroke. Contrary to what the title may suggest, the reader will become aware of the limitations of physical examination in this setting but will not learn new techniques for the assessment of stroke patients.

644. Guarino JR. Auscultatory percussion of the head. *Br Med J.* 1982; 284:1075-7.

The data herein suggest that finger and stethoscope are nearly the equivalent of computed tomography in detecting such masses as subdural hematomas. They may outperform imaging in locating *old* strokes. Simple but rigorous experimental support, but issues of bias in clinical use remain thorny.

645. Haerer AF. *DeJong's the Neurologic Examination.* **5th ed. Philadelphia: JB Lippincott; 1992.**

The encyclopedic final court of law on the neuroanatomic bases of neurologic signs, their elicitation, and interpretation.

646. Goldberg S. *The 4-Minute Neurologic Exam (An Answer to the "Neuro WNL" Problem).* Miami: MedMaster; 1987.

Despite its perhaps excessively short format, this booklet offers a rational neurologic examination that could be easily performed in the allotted 4 minutes. Might be useful to third-year medical students who are so often overwhelmed by standard texts.

647. Landau WM. Strategy, tactics, and accuracy in neurological evaluation [Editorial]. *Ann Neurol.* **1990;28:86-7.**

A recognized senior clinician offers some analysis of how to generate and test hypotheses in this area.

648. Massey EW, Scherokman B. Soft neurologic signs. *Postgrad Med.* 1981; 70:66-70.

Reviews soft neurologic signs in terms that are understandable and germane to non-neurologists, explaining which are significant and when. Even a Babinski sign can become "soft" in certain contexts!

649. Medical Research Council. *Aids to the Investigation of Peripheral Nerve Injuries.* **London: Her Majesty's Stationery Office; 1972.**

Straightforward, understandable, and amazing: a simple bedside means to test the innervation of almost every muscle one can think of.

650. Ziegler DK. Is the neurologic examination becoming obsolete? *Neurology.* **1985;35:559.**

The answer is easy to predict; the road to reaching the answer is an interesting one. The suggestions in this article for re-evaluating old signs in relation to fancy new technologies resemble those of Nardone (*see* references 11 and 12).

History

651. Blau JN. How to take a history of head or facial pain. *Br Med J.* **1982; 285:1249-51.**

Generalizes to include advice on effective characterization of any symptom, not just headache alone.

652. Simms RW, Goldenberg DL. Symptoms mimicking neurologic disorders in fibromyalgia syndrome. *J Rheumatol.* **1988;15:1271-3.**

In a rheumatologic referral practice, the prevalence of paresthesias in the fibromyalgia syndrome was greater than 80%. They were often intermittent and correlated at times with the course of other fibromyalgia symptoms.

Autonomic nervous system assessment

653. Korpelainen JT, Sotaniemi KA, Myllyla VV. Asymmetrical skin temperature in ischemic stroke. *Stroke.* **1995;26:1543-7.**

Using technology, this study shows that both arms and legs contralateral to cerebral hemispheric infarctions are cooler than their opposites, perhaps from hyperhidrosis. This phenomenon tends to parallel pyramidal tract signs, starts acutely, and persists at 6 months after stroke, and the patient is often aware of and dislikes a sense of coldness in the paretic limb. Owing to ipsilateral *hypo*hidrosis in Wallenberg's syndrome, the same temperature differential occurs in some brain stem strokes. Uses a very youthful sample for a stroke study: mean age of 54 years, with the oldest patient only 69 years old. Correlation with the methods in reference 655 would be of interest.

654. Schwartzman RJ, McLellan TL. Reflex sympathetic dystrophy: a review. *Arch Neurol.* **1987;44:555-61.**

Ranges well beyond the physical findings. The nonmusculoskeletal specialist can profitably extract the symptoms and signs from this article.

655. Tsementzis SA, Hitchcock ER. The spoon test: a simple bedside test for assessing sudomotor autonomic failure. *J Neurol Neurosurg Psychiatry.* **1985;48:378-80.**

Describes how, to seek localized autonomic dysfunction, the examiner should hold a soup spoon between thumb and forefinger, with the curved surface down, and draw it slowly across the skin without supporting its weight. It will move too easily and unopposed if sympathetic sweating is lost, and more stickily if function is intact. Precise localization of sudomotor dysfunction will not correspond to somatosensory deficit.

Cerebral function

(*see also* Mental status)

656. Anonymous. Forgotten symptoms and primitive signs. *Lancet.* **1987; 1:841-2.**

Asserts that grasp, palmomental, and glabellar signs, and some other symptoms and signs appear to have little or no diagnostic or localizing value in most settings. "Hallowed" parts of the armamentarium that are unable to earn their keep need not be perpetuated.

657. Damasio AR. Aphasia (Medical Progress). *N Engl J Med.* **1992;326:531-40.**

Erudite, at times overwhelming, discussion of the details and nuances of aphasia.

658. Jenkyn LR, Walsh DB, Culver CM, Reeves AG. Clinical signs in diffuse cerebral dysfunction. *J Neurol Neurosurg Psychiatry.* **1977;40:956-66.**

This article is part of a continuing search for combinations of neurologic findings that will predict dementia, parallel to the search for equally prognostically and diagnostically potent findings from mental status testing.

659. Thomas RJ. Blinking and the release reflexes: are they clinically useful? *J Am Geriatr Soc.* **1994;42:609-13.**

Good review of the mechanisms and clinical significance of frontal release signs, despite the contention of others that they are obsolescent.

Cranial nerves

660. Ruffin R, Rachootin P. Gag reflex in disease [Letter]. *Chest.* **1987;92:1130.**

Discusses how, in a simple prevalence study, many patients without neurologic disease lacked a gag reflex. The clinical significance and even the permanence or transience of this dysfunction are unknown.

Meningeal signs

661. Callaham M. Fulminant bacterial meningitis without meningeal signs. *Ann Emerg Med.* **1989;18:90-3.**

The unfortunate lack of sensitivity of meningeal signs in infancy and old age is widely recognized. Less familiar are instances of false-negative examinations that occur *after* infancy and *before* old age. If acute bacterial meningitis is suspected, one should not be deterred from lumbar puncture by the absence of meningeal signs.

662. Verghese A, Gallemore G. Kernig's and Brudzinski's signs revisited. *Rev Infect Dis*. 1987;9:1187-92.

Superb review that begins with re-examination of the original papers on these topics and proceeds to a discussion of the relevant function of the signs for today's clinician.

Motor examination including abnormal involuntary movements

663. Alter M. The digiti quinti sign of mild hemiparesis. *Neurology*. 1973; 23:503-5.

A description of this sign: the fifth (little) finger has less cortical representation than the other fingers and is slightly abducted contralateral to an old precentral infarct when the hands are held forward. Follow-up and validation studies are needed.

664. Barnes TRE. A rating scale for drug-induced akathisia. *Br J Psychiatry*. 1989;154:672-6.

Discusses a version of this scale that has fallen into relative disuse compared to the regular AIMS (abnormal involuntary movements scale), but is worthy of review and occasional application.

665. Beatty RM, Fowler FD, Hanson EJ Jr. The abducted arm as a sign of ruptured cervical disc. *Neurosurgery*. 1987;21:731-2.

Describes how when a lateral cervical disc protrusion is present, abduction of the ipsilateral arm may relieve the pain and serve as a clue to the diagnosis.

666. Csuka M, McCarty DJ. Simple method for measurement of lower extremity muscle strength. *Am J Med*. 1985;78:77-81.

The authors describe their "timed stands" test: the examiner measures how long it takes for the patient to rise from a sitting position on a standardized chair to a standing position 10 times. This is a simple and reproducible test that can be used as an objective serial measurement of lower extremity strength, and it is especially useful for longitudinal follow-up of patients with neuromuscular disorders.

667. Dyck P. The stoop-test in lumbar entrapment radiculopathy. *Spine*. 1979;4:89-92.

Describes a version of the bicycle test (*see* reference 595): the examiner has the patient stand upright and walk briskly down a straight corridor. With impingement on neural structures as in lumbar spinal stenosis, buttock and limb pain will develop. Continuing the walk worsens the pain, then weakness develops. This is eased when the patient stoops while continuing to walk but is worsened when he or she stops and stands upright. Sitting down and leaning forward eliminates the symptoms.

668. **Munetz MR, Benjamin S. How to examine patients using the abnormal involuntary movement scale.** *Hosp Comm Psychiatr.* **1988;39:1172-7.**

Describes a simple series of neurologic observations of the whole patient, as well as a few questions to ask about the patient's awareness of his or her movements and about the state of oral function. The test is currently done most often by nursing staff. The non-neurologist, nonpsychiatrist is well advised to take the few minutes required to learn how to administer, record, and interpret the scale.

669. **Nelson KR, Bicknell JM. Oblique pectoral crease and "scapular hump" in shoulder contour are signs of trapezius muscle weakness.** *J Neurol Neurosurg Psychiatry.* **1987;50:1082-3.**

Discusses how downward and forward displacement of the shoulder and elevation of the superior angle of the scapula produce these signs in trapezius weakness, with or without dysfunction of other nearby muscles.

670. **Ono K, Ebara S, Fuji T, et al. Myelopathy hand: new clinical signs of cervical cord damage.** *J Bone Joint Surg Br.* **1987;69-B:215-9.**

Discusses how with injury to the cervical cord from spondylosis, abduction of the fifth finger can occur that is similar to the digiti quinti sign; in more advanced cases, fixed flexion of the metacarpophalangeal joints of the three ulnar fingers occurs, then loss of ability to flex and extend all fingers rapidly in concert occur. This does not occur in radiculopathy in the same area. Common bedside tests exclude another possible mimic, ulnar neuropathy.

671. **Reinfeld H, Louis S. Unilateral asterixis: clinical significance of the sign.** *N Y State J Med.* **1983;83:206-8.**

Describes how rather than signifying metabolic encephalopathy as does conventional bilateral asterixis, this variant indicates a structural lesion, often frontoparietal but sometimes midbrain, thalamic, or other. Adds the fine points that opposition to gravity is essential for eliciting asterixis (i.e., asterixis cannot be reliably elicited if the patient is supine and gravity is helping to keep the wrists extended); that the latency is 3 to 30 seconds; and that asterixis can also be prominent at the ankles.

672. Massey EW, Goodman JC, Stewart C, Brannon WL. Unilateral asterixis: motor integrative dysfunction in focal vascular disease. *Neurology.* 1979;29:1180-2 (misprinted on abstract as 1188-1190).

Shows that unilateral asterixis is perhaps more common than one might suspect. Three cases were caused by strokes in and about the internal capsule; these were transiently associated with mild ipsilateral hemiparesis.

673. Santamaria J, Graus F, Genis D. Bilateral asterixis in unilateral subdural hematoma. *J Neurol.* 1983;229:87-9.

Describes a single exception to the rule that unilaterality is structural and that bilaterality is functional (metabolic). Speculates that deep midline structures may be involved.

674. Wee AS. Unilateral asterixis: case report and comments. *Eur Neurol.* 1986;25:208-11.

A reminder that when it is bilateral, asterixis can be asynchronous and of unequal prominence.

675. **Riley TL, Ray WF, Massey EW. Gait mechanisms: asymmetry of arm motion in normal subjects. *Mil Med.* 1977;141:467-8.**

Establishes that this finding is not a soft sign of hemiparesis or of basal nucleus dysfunction (parkinsonism).

676. **Sanes JN, Hallett M. Limb positioning and magnitude of essential tremor and other pathological tremors. *Mov Disord.* 190;5:304-9.**

Using a piezoelectric wrist accelerometer to quantitate tremor, the authors noted an increase in the intensity of the tremor when the patient's hand was closer to the face. This effect was more prominent in cases of pathologic tumor than in those of essential tremor.

677. **Siegler EL, Beck LH. Stiffness: a pathophysiologic approach to diagnosis and treatment. *J Gen Intern Med.* 1989;4:533-40.**

Descriptive article with detailed, specific advice on highest-utility features in the physical examination, followed by a discussion of several common causes of the symptom and sign.

678. **Wallace GB, Newton RW. Gower's sign revisited. *Arch Dis Child Br.* 1989;64:1317-9.**

Discusses one of the two variants—namely, rolling prone before arising; persistence of this behavior in a child at the age of 3 years calls for neurologic assessment.

Muscle stretch reflexes, plantars, and related findings

679. **Goode DJ, Van Hoven J. Loss of patellar and Achilles tendon reflexes in classical ballet dancers [Letter]. *Arch Neurol.* 1982;39:323.**

Discusses how ballet dancers may have decreased or absent plantar reflexes. Possible mechanisms are unclear.

680. **Grant R. The neurological assault on the great toe (1893–1911). *Scot Med J.* 1987;32:57-9.**

A historical exploration that helps one get all of those eponyms straight and, more importantly, places them in context.

681. Healton EB, Savage DG, Brust JC, et al. Neurologic aspects of cobalamin deficiency. *Medicine.* **1991;70:229-45.**

Discusses how patients with neuropathic symptoms despite normal neurologic examination are common in this setting. If the examiner does not consider the symptoms psychogenic, measurement of the serum level of vitamin B_{12} is warranted no matter what the hematocrit value and mean corpuscular volume are.

682. Schwartz RS, Morris JG, Crimmins D, et al. A comparison of two methods of eliciting the ankle jerk. *Aust N Z J Med.* **1990;20:116-9.**

Describes how a tap on the sole of the foot seems to be as effective for evaluation of the Achilles reflex as the more widely used tap on the Achilles tendon.

683. Shimizu T, Shimada H, Shirakura K. Scapulohumeral reflex (Shimizu): its clinical significance and testing maneuver. *Spine.* **1993;18:2182-90.**

Description of a case series to substantiate the use of the scapulohumeral reflex (Shimizu variant technique) to detect cervical myelopathy above the C3 vertebral body level. The reflex is of value only when hyperactive and bilateral. It consists of elevation of the scapula or humerus or both upon tapping the tip of the scapula or the acromion. One can become familiar with the abnormal response by eliciting it unilaterally in stroke patients.

684. Wise MP, Blunt S, Lane RJM. Neurological presentations of hypothyroidism: the importance of slow relaxing reflexes. *J R Soc Med.* **1995; 88:272-4.**

The value of slow relaxing deep tendon reflexes is illustrated by three case reports.

Sensory examination

685. Caplan LR. The small corks test: a rapid sensory screening test. *JAMA.* **1981;246:1341-2.**

Describes a test in which the examiner takes four corks of graded size ranging from 1 to 2 cm in height and in maximum diameter and places them in the patient's hand for him or her to study, while the patient keeps his or her eyes closed. The examiner encourages the patient to manipulate the corks, but only with the one hand that holds the corks. The examiner then asks the patient to hand him the largest cork, the second-largest cork, and so on, until all are returned. Mental dysfunction or severe motor problems preclude the test. In persons without mental dysfunction or severe motor problems, it has high sensitivity, specificity, and speed in detecting sensory dysfunction.

686. **Nelson KR. Use new pins for each neurologic examination [Letter].** *N Engl J Med.* **1986;314:581.**

Discusses one means of avoiding transmission of HIV and hepatitis B. Previous and equally valid pleas for this simple and necessary behavioral alteration have been made to prevent the transmission of conventional and slow viruses.

Other issues and specific conditions

687. **Betts T. Pseudoseizures: seizures that are not epilepsy.** *Lancet.* **1990; 336:163-4.**

Discusses how some pseudoseizures are such close mimics that even an experienced neurologist watching them may be misled. Makes a clear case for the need for simultaneous brain wave recording and videotaping in the most difficult cases.

688. **Hemachudha T, Phanthumchinda K, Phanuphak P, Manutsathit S. Myoedema as a clinical sign in paralytic rabies [Letter].** *Lancet.* **1987; 1:1210.**

Describes how when the muscle is tapped, it rapidly swells up. Previously, this sign was thought of predominantly in relation to hypothyroidism and malnutrition.

689. **Louis S. A bedside test for determining the sub-types of vascular headache.** *Headache.* **1981;21:87-8.**

Discusses how this test is most commonly used in migraine evaluation. Ninety-five percent of migraines have an external carotid vasodilatory origin and 5% of migraines have an internal carotid origin. The examiner has the patient perform a Valsalva maneuver, which should reduce any vascular headache, with resumption of pain a few seconds after release; this maneuver is repeated with the superficial temporal arteries compressed by the examiner's fingers. If the pain does not increase on release of the Valsalva maneuver but only upon release of the temporal arteries thereafter, it is of external carotid origin. Somewhat analogous to the bruit characterization in reference 429.

Mental Status and Psychiatric Evaluation

690. **Anthony JC, LeResche L, Niaz U, et al. Limits of the 'Mini-Mental State' as a screening test for dementia and delirium among hospital patients.** *Psych Med.* **1982;12:397-408.**

Discusses intrinsic problems with the sensitivity of the test (e.g., false-negatives in highly educated persons) and its specificity (e.g., false-positives in persons with sensory or motor impairment, independent of their true cognitive capacity).

691. **Geldmacher DS, Whitehouse PJ. Evaluation of dementia.** *N Engl J Med.* **1996;335:330-6.**

Useful also for initial detection of dementia and for evaluation of patients with suspected rather than confirmed dementia (hence its inclusion in this portion of the bibliography and not in the section on special-needs patients with dementia and mental retardation). Table 1 of this article, the supplemental bedside mental status examinations to assess possible or confirmed dementia, is particularly pragmatic for incorporation into daily practice.

692. **Jacoby R. Loss of memory and concentration.** *Br J Hosp Med.* **1985; 33:32-4.**

Concise work on the separation of dementia from pseudodementia and organic causes.

693. **Molloy DW, Alemayehu E, Roberts R. Reliability of a standardized Mini-Mental State Examination compared with the traditional Mini-Mental State Examination.** *Am J Psychiatry.* **1991;148:102-5.**

Discusses the way in which modifications simplify administration of the test, make it routine, decrease the time it takes to complete the test, and render it more accurate. To request the modified test, readers need to contact the senior author: D.W. Molloy, M.B., McMaster University Clinic, Henderson General Hospital, Department of Medicine, 711 Concession Street, Hamilton, Ontario, Canada L8V 1C3.

694. Strain JJ, Fulop G. Screening devices for cognitive capacity [Editorial]. *Ann Intern Med*. 1987;107:583-5.

Editorial published with the neurobehavioral cognitive status examination test report. Includes a fine general discussion on cognitive-mental status testing instruments that can be used by the internist (as distinct from those that only the psychiatrist or psychologist uses). Many of the comments and caveats apply equally well to more familiar screening devices such as the Folstein Mini-Mental Status Examination.

695. Strub RL, Black FW. *The Mental Status Examination in Neurology*. 3rd ed. Philadelphia: FA Davis; 1983.

Includes listings and descriptions of mental status test and findings that are of importance not only to psychiatrists and neurologists but also to every nonpsychiatric clinician.

696. Tombaugh TN, McIntyre NJ. The Mini-Mental State Examination: a comprehensive review. *J Am Geriatr Soc*. 1992;40:922-35.

Sober, expert, and highly referenced review by nonphysicians. The practical suggestions at the end of the article include the following: not basing a diagnosis of dementia on this test exclusively; classifying mild cognitive impairment by a score of 18–23; not using the test if the patient has less than an eighth-grade education or is not fluent in English; testing serial 7's *and* backwards-spelling of WORLD, and using the better performance of the two to score; offering the polysyllabic words "apple, penny, and table" for the three-item registration and recall; and changing the county and hospital floor items. Unfortunately, the review does not incorporate the excellent suggestions of Molloy and colleagues (reference 693).

697. Watson YI, Arfken CL, Birge SJ. Clock completion: an objective screening method for dementia. *J Am Geriatr Soc*. 1993;41:1235-40.

Simplified scoring: the patient should not be asked to put in the hands on the clock; the examiner should simply count the number of items (not digits) in the left upper quadrant of the clock, counting those that fall on any quadrant line as lying clockwise to the line. Of course, drawing three items in the quadrant is the correct response (i.e., normal); any other figure is incorrect (i.e., abnormal).

698. Sunderland T, Hill JL, Mellow AM, et al. Clock drawing in Alzheimer's disease: a novel measure of dementia severity. *J Am Geriatr Soc*. 1989;37:725-9.

Describes a somewhat different test than that described in reference 697, also exceptionally well thought out.

699. Wolf-Klein GP, Silverstone FA, Levy AP, et al. Screening for Alzheimer's disease by clock drawing. *J Am Geriatr Soc*. 1989;37:730-4.

Describes an easily performed maneuver that helped the authors classify cognitive function, in conjunction with other standard mental status examinations. As an exploration of spatial orientation and temporoparietal function, the test may assist recognition of primary degenerative dementia at a stage in which, or in a host in whom, linguistic deficits have not yet become manifest.

700. Weller MP. Neuropsychiatric symptoms following bismuth intoxication. *Postgrad Med J*. 1988;64:308-10.

Discusses neurotic and neuropathic-myelopathic symptoms that abated when chronic "therapeutic" ingestion was stopped. With the increasing popularity of bismuth subsalicylate for the treatment of *Helicobacter pylori*–induced peptic disease, the syndrome needs to be kept in mind.

Mental status findings in non-neuropsychiatric disease

701. Medvei VC, Cattell WR. Mental symptoms presenting in phaeochromocytoma: a case report and review. *J R Soc Med*. 1988;81:550-1.

Discusses an association that the first author has explored for four decades.

702. Regan WM. Thyrotoxicosis manifested as mania. *South Med J*. 1988; 81:1460-1.

We all need to be reminded of the occurrence of physical disease presenting in a psychiatric guise (even of so classical an example as the one described in this article).

Geriatric Bedside Assessment

General material

703. Kamal A, Brocklehurst JC. *Color Atlas of Geriatric Medicine.* **2nd ed. St. Louis: Mosby Year–Book; 1991.**

Includes lively illustrations in a work co-authored by an eminent authority in the field.

704. Libow L. Evaluating the elderly patient: some overlooked aspects. *Geriatrics.* **1987;42:18, 20.**

Includes a two-page introduction to functional assessment and a discussion of the two chief complaints (those of the patient and of the family), advance directives, and other key issues.

705. Schneiderman H. Physical examination of the aged patient. *Conn Med.* **1993;57:317-24.**

General review and a description of several specific techniques. Includes material on history-taking as well as the title subject.

History

706. Buchsbaum DG, Buchanan RG, Welsh J, et al. Screening for drinking disorders in the elderly using the CAGE questionnaire. *J Am Geriatr Soc.* **1992;40:662-5.**

Extends the validation of this useful instrument to elderly persons and describes applying analysis of receiver operating characteristic (ROC) curves to provide multiple possible cut-offs, each with its own positive predictive value, instead of using a "one-score-fits-all" approach. Important use of Bayesian theory: higher cut-offs should be used for lower-prevalence groups, such as women. The tables offer a more useful source of data than the ROC curves, which are not well understood by most clinicians.

707. **Clinch D, Banerjee AK, Ostick G. Absence of abdominal pain in elderly patients with peptic ulcer.** *Age Ageing.* **1984;13:120-3.**

In this study, one third of elderly patients with endoscopically established ulcers had no pain. This study has methodologic and conceptual problems.

708. **Davis PB, Robins LN. History-taking in the elderly with and without cognitive impairment: how useful is it?** *J Am Geriatr Soc.* **1989;37:249-55.**

Discusses how even when the patient has considerable brain dysfunction, one may be able to elicit meaningful information regarding current symptoms. The history should not employ collateral informants exclusively.

709. **Greene MS, Majerovitz SD, Adelman RD, Rizzo C. The effects of the presence of a third person on the physician–older patient medical interview.** *J Am Geriatr Soc.* **1994;42:413-9.**

Discusses the way in which a third person may divert attention from the patient, who is frequently excluded from conversation. A very important article on vital, previously untouched ground; a great deal of additional research is needed.

710. **Howard R, Turner G. Why don't we take adequate drinking histories from elderly admissions?** *Br J Addict.* **1989;84:1374-5.**

The frequency of alcoholism and alcohol-related health problems in elderly persons seems to be under-recognized. Consider the real story: 10% or so of elderly patients admitted to the hospital have health problems that are alcohol related. Routine exploration of this issue is needed.

711. **Steel K. History taking from elderly patients.** *Hosp Pract.* **1985; 20(5A):70-1.**

Compact, insightful statement of the many problems involved in history taking from elderly patients. Offers practical and straightforward remedies.

General appearance, functional assessment, and falls

712. **Cooney LM Jr. Assessment of immobility in the elderly.** *Conn Med.* **1993;57:281-6.**

A very lucid short course on the importance of testing mobility function by physical examination and on interpreting the results, in the areas of sit-to-stand and sit-to-sit transfers, static sitting balance, safety awareness, gait, bracing, and assistive devices.

713. **Lachs MS, Feinstein AR, Cooney LM Jr, et al. A simple procedure for general screening for functional disability in elderly patients.** *Ann Intern Med.* 1990;112:699-706.

This highly user-friendly article offers 10 extremely straightforward and quick screening tests in 10 important areas. It also provides interpretation and describes a follow-up step to take for any impairment that is found.

714. **Mathias S, Nayak USL, Isaacs B. Balance in elderly patients: the "get up and go" test.** *Arch Phys Med Rehabil.* 1986;67:387-9.

Describes a test in which the patient sits in a straight-backed chair and is then asked to rise, to stand still for a moment, to walk 3 meters, to turn back, walk to the chair, turn again, and sit. Standardized grading is used. The test compared favorably with laboratory assessment of balance. An important antecedent to the work of Tinetti (reference 741) and particularly to that of Guralnik (references 736 and 737).

715. **Pines A, Levo Y. Straight or oblique? [Letter].** *J Am Geriatr Soc.* 1989; 37:1004.

Discusses how patients sprawled diagonally across the bed seem more often markedly demented or psychiatrically impaired compared with straight-lying peers.

716. **Rousseau P. The lateral slump sign as an indicator of infection in the elderly.** *J Am Geriatr Soc.* 1992;40:1024-5.

Describes how a single demented parkinsonian patient with a urinary tract infection slumped to the right, became unwontedly tractable, stayed indoors, and lost his craving for tobacco. All of these behaviors reversed after antibiotic therapy. Slumping to one side is a nonspecific indicator of a change in overall health and is not by any means limited to infection.

717. Becker WG. The lateral slump sign [Letter]. *J Am Geriatr Soc.* 1993;41:344.

Seeks to extend Rousseau's observations with a clinical anecdote and by tying it in with the more general phenomenon of reduced mobility as a nonspecific indicator of disease in elderly persons. By contrast, lying obliquely across the bed has been associated with permanent cognitive loss and not with acute illness (*see* reference 715).

718. **Schneiderman H, Pitegoff G. Nasal fracture and facial ecchymoses from violent fall, and falls assessment.** *Consultant.* 1995;35:1701-5.

Describes simple bedside tests that should be done in these patients, such as orthostatic pulse and blood pressure measurement. Emphasizes avoiding the syncope work-up in the large fraction of patients who have sustained falls that did not result from loss of consciousness.

719. **Winograd CH, Lemsky CM, Nevitt MC, et al. Development of a physical performance and mobility examination.** *J Am Geriatr Soc.* **1994;42:743-9.**

Discusses a rapid six-activity test designed to determine mobility function to yield insights that are complementary to those from self-reported activities of daily living. Very careful methodology. The applicability, convenience, and predictive value of the test in populations other than the hospitalized aged are still being evaluated.

Vital signs

720. **Cunha BA. Fever of unknown origin in the elderly.** *Geriatrics.* **1982; 37:30-44.**

This complex subset of a challenging entity still requires, above all other investigations, a lengthy, specific interview and examination.

721. **Howell TH. Oral temperature range in old age.** *Gerontologia Clinica.* **1975;17:133-6.**

This simple study addresses quite nicely some sources of artifact. Lack of controlling for oral intake may have artifactually lowered mouth temperature.

722. **McFadden JP, Price RC, Eastwood HD, Briggs RS. Raised respiratory rate in elderly patients: a valuable physical sign.** *Br Med J.* **1982;284:626-7.**

Retrospective review showed that the respiratory rate often started climbing before an acute illness became "differentiated" and thus recognizable as a respiratory tract infection.

Head and giant cell arteritis

723. **Larson TS, Hall S, Hepper NG, Hunder GG. Respiratory tract symptoms as a clue to giant cell arteritis.** *Ann Intern Med.* **1984;101:594-7.**

Discusses how cough, sore throat, and hoarseness are prominent in nearly one tenth of cases of giant cell arteritis. There is some overlap with symptoms previously classified as carotid arteritis and with other and more conventional forms of both upper and lower respiratory tract disease.

724. **Pye M. Lingual and scalp infarction as a manifestation of giant cell arteritis: delay in diagnosis leading to blindness [Letter].** *J Rheumatol.* **1988;15:1597-8.**

Includes extraordinary photographs, along with a recounting of an autopsy study that showed surprisingly frequent involvement of the lingual arteries in this condition.

Eye examination

725. Roederer GO, Bouthillier D, Davignon J. Xanthelasma palpebrarum and corneal arcus in octogenarians [Letter]. *N Engl J Med.* **1987;317:1740.**

Discusses a simple idea but includes some unfamiliar material about apolipoprotein E phenotypes. It seems that the signs do *not* have predictive value for vascular disease in this population.

Ear and hearing assessment

726. Lichtenstein MJ, Bess FH, Logan SA. Validation of screening tools for identifying hearing-impaired elderly in primary care. *JAMA.* **1988;259:2875-8.**

Discusses how an audioscope and a simple questionnaire were combined to improve the sensitivity and specificity of identifying hearing deficits.

727. Uhlmann RF, Rees TS, Psaty BM, Duckert LG. Validity and reliability of auditory screening tests in demented and non-demented older adults. *J Gen Intern Med.* **1989;4:90-5.**

This study shows considerable test-retest reliability in demented persons, in some cases exceeding the corresponding figures for nondemented persons! Shows that simple auditory evaluation can therefore be meaningful and can lead to an intervention that may enhance quality of life.

Oral examination

728. Gordon SR, Jahnigen DW. Oral assessment of the edentulous elderly patient. *J Am Geriatr Soc.* **1983;31:797-801.**

Because such persons see their dentists rarely if at all, guidelines are provided for the physician to examine the mouth and dentures and to counsel patients on oral health in the setting of edentia.

Breasts

729. Baines CJ. Physical examination of the breasts in screening for breast cancer. *J Gerontol.* **1992;47 (Special issue):63-7.**

Reviews studies that claim that clinical breast examination adds almost nothing to mammography in a screening program, and notes that one problem that occurred in at least one center was inept physical examination technique, "consisting only of palpation of the four breast quadrants with the cupped hand." Gives in detail the longer but diagnostically more effective standardized examination procedure taught to the nurse-clinicians of the Canadian National Breast Screening Study (which is also the subject of reference 298).

Heart

730. **Wong M, Tei C, Shah PM. Degenerative calcific valvular disease and systolic murmurs in the elderly.** *J Am Geriatr Soc.* **1983;31:156-63.**

Documents the hemodynamic innocence of this common entity. The assertion of the propensity of valves with this murmur to infective endocarditis is unsupported.

Mental status evaluation

731. **Braekhus A, Laake K, Engedahl K. A low, "normal" score on the minimental state examination predicts development of dementia after three years.** *J Am Geriatr Soc.* **1995;43:656-61.**

A very provocative Norwegian study. By the authors' own account as well as by the reader's judgment, this is far from the last word on the predictive value of scores that, albeit previously in the normal range, lie at its lower end.

732. **Heeren TJ, Lagaay AM, Beek WC, et al. Reference values for the Mini-Mental State Examination (MMSE) in octo- and non-agenarians.** *J Am Geriatric Soc.* **1990;38:1093-6.**

Shows that, although these reference values are lower than in normal 60-year-olds, one can often use them to distinguish dementia from nondementia with good certainty nonetheless.

733. **Moss R, D'Amico S, Maletta G. Mental dysfunction as a sign of organic illness in the elderly.** *Geriatrics.* **1987;42:35-42.**

A discussion of the widely accepted concept that the brain is often the most tenuously compensated organ in elderly persons and is prone to dysfunction from any systemic derangement. That is the basis of the old saying, "If you find a newly confused old person without an evident explanation, look for pneumonia."

734. **Shreve ST, Schneiderman H. Dementia-associated visuospatial cognitive dysfunction demonstrated by the draw-a-clock test.** *Consultant.* **1994; 34:1301-3.**

A brief, illustrated discussion of the draw-a-clock test, an easily administered bedside evaluation that is complementary to the Mini-Mental State Examination by assessing a different domain of cognition.

735. Mendez MF, Ala T, Underwood KL. Development of scoring criteria for the clock drawing task in Alzheimer's disease. *J Am Geriatr Soc.* 1992;40:1095-9.

This easy-to-administer test complements the language-preponderant assessment of the Mini-Mental State Examination. The criteria of Mendez's group have been superseded by those of Watson and associates (reference 697), but this article deserves review for its additional insights.

Mobility, musculoskeletal assessment, and gait

736. Guralnik JM, Ferrucci L, Simonsick EM, et al. Lower-extremity function in persons over the age of 70 years as a predictor of subsequent disability. *N Engl J Med.* **1995;332:556-61.**

In this study, a group of community-dwelling elderly persons who self-reported ability to walk a long distance and to climb stairs were given a battery of simple physical-diagnostic tests, including assessments of stance and balance, timed walking of 8 feet at a normal pace, and timed rising from a hair and sitting back down five times in succession. Those with the poorest scores had a markedly increased risk of disability on 4-year follow-up. The tests may thus identify a preclinical stage of mobility dysfunction.

737. Guralnik JM, Simonsick EM, Ferrucci L, et al. A short physical performance battery assessing lower extremity function: association with self-reported disability and prediction of mortality and nursing home admission. *J Gerontol: Med Sci.* 1994;49:M85-M94.

The conclusions and issues of this study are similar to those of the *New England Journal of Medicine* report (reference 736), but this earlier study has additional methodologic detail and discussion.

738. Schneiderman H, Bellantonio S. Kyphosis due to osteoporotic compression fractures of thoracic vertebrae. *Consultant.* **1996;36:507-9.**

Discussion of the role of physical examination to suggest, in visually accessible areas, what is occurring internally.

739. Sudarsky L. Geriatrics: gait disorders in the elderly. *N Engl J Med.* **1990;322:1441-6.**

See combined review in reference 740.

740. Caranasos GJ, Israel R. Gait disorders in the elderly. *Hosp Pract.* 1991;26:67-70, 75, 79-82, 91-2, 94.

Practical reviews on the approach to gait abnormalities in elderly persons, with a focus on diagnosis.

741. Tinetti ME, Ginter SF. Identifying mobility dysfunctions in elderly patients: standard neuromuscular examination or direct assessment? *JAMA.* **1988;259:1190-3.**

Discusses how a simple series of maneuvers correlates better with function at home than does the traditional (and more time-consuming) physical examination of individual muscles, nerves, and joints.

Neurologic examination

742. **Brown RA, Lawson DA, Leslie GC, Part NJ. Observations on the applicability of the Wartenberg pendulum test to healthy, elderly subjects.** *J Neurol Neurosurg Psychiatry.* **1988;51:1171-7.**

The test consists of letting a passively extended knee drop, and recording the arcs subtended until it comes to rest. As with the following study (reference 743), has minimal applicability to routine clinical practice. Computer analysis is required to interpret the test result, precluding bedside use.

743. Brown RA, Lawson DA, Leslie GC, et al. Does the Wartenberg pendulum test differentiate quantitatively between spasticity and rigidity? A study in elderly stroke and parkinsonian patients. *J Neurol Neurosurg Psychiatry.* 1988;51:1178-86.

The answer to the title question is "possibly," if the computerized system used by the investigators is taken into account. For practical purposes, the test cannot be endorsed as better than any other method for evaluating muscle tone.

744. **Gray CS, Walker A. The plantar response: caution in the elderly.** *Br J Hosp Med.* **1989;42:105-6.**

Brave case reports of damage to the sole of the foot and the anterior shin. Considering the frequency of neuropathy, ischemia, venous insufficiency, and fragile skin in elderly persons, the surprise is that this does not occur more often.

745. **Impallomeni M, Flynn MD, Kenny RA, et al. The elderly and their ankle jerks.** *Lancet.* **1984;1:670-2.**

Using modifications in the timing of doing the test (second hospital day, rather than on admission) and in technique, the authors found almost no areflexia that could be ascribed to age alone without neurologic disease. We have been unable to duplicate these exciting results.

746. **O'Keeffe ST, Smith T, Valacio R, et al. A comparison of two techniques for ankle jerk assessment in elderly subjects.** *Lancet.* **1994;344:1619-20.**

Describes a technique in which the plantar surface is tapped with the hammer, while the fingers of the examiner's free hand cushion the blow. Possibly more reproducible than the familiar blow to tendo Achillis. The results are imperfect and the methods can be faulted—for example, because of the absence of a Jendrassik reinforcement to bring out lesser responses.

747. O'Brien MD. Ankle jerk assessment [Letter]. *Lancet.* 1995;345:331.

Claims that there is higher consistency because the plantar tap is less sensitive.

748. Pryor JP. Ankle jerk assessment [Letter]. *Lancet.* 1995;345:331.

Advocates eliciting the ankle jerk in men in the left lateral decubitus position, with hips and knees flexed, just after performing rectal examination.

749. Puxty JA, Fox RA, Horan MA. The frequency of physical signs usually attributed to meningeal irritation in elderly patients. *J Am Geriatr Soc.* **1983;31:590-2.**

Discusses how many elderly persons who are examined when perfectly healthy have nuchal rigidity, a Kernig sign, or a Brudzinski sign; demented elderly persons had the highest prevalence. This sign thus may potentially mislead the physician working up a fever or a mental status change.

750. Walshe TM. Neurologic examination of the elderly patient: signs of normal aging. *Postgrad Med.* **1987;81:375-8.**

A concise review, which could lead to avoiding testing vibratory sensation in screening: only position sense deficits point to posterior column dysfunction, because vibratory sensation can decline with normal aging.

Genital and rectal examinations

751. Clinical Practice Committee. Screening for cervical carcinoma in elderly women. *J Am Geriatr Soc.* **1989;37:885-7.**

The oft-repeated dictum that Pap smears are not necessary in women older than 70 years has no scientific base unless the patient has had multiple negative tests in the previous decade. Use of a saline-moistened swab introduced into the cervical canal is more necessary than in younger women because the squamocolumnar junction tends to recede with age.

752. Dumesic DA. Pelvic examination: what to focus on in menopausal women. *Consultant.* **1996;36:39-46.**

A short and satisfactorily illustrated review of the topic, including practical information on putting the appropriately apprehensive patient at ease, on speculum sizes, and on the endocervical cytology brush. The focus on taking biopsies oneself may not appeal to internists.

753. Smith RG, Lewis S. The relationship between digital rectal examination and abdominal radiographs in elderly patients. *Age Ageing.* **1990; 19:142-3.**

Shows that one can have a full rectum by digital examination and an empty colon by radiography! Conversely and more familiarly, an empty rectum on digital exploration does not exclude proximal impaction. The authors conclude that radiographs are needed to assess possible fecal impaction but unfortunately make no correlation with conventional abdominal palpation. Until that additional element is tested, the role of abdominal radiographs is undecided. In the meantime, their correlation of soft rectal feces with cecal fecal loading was stronger than that of hard feces in the rectum!

754. Speas CK, Gallup DC, Gallup DG. Hematocolpos in elderly women. *South Med J.* **1993;86:815-8.**

Discusses how this condition can be acquired when synechiae close off egress from the vagina and uterus, particularly after surgery or radiotherapy to the area.

Human Immunodeficiency Virus
(HIV) Infection: Bedside Assessment

General material

755. **Adams F. The "sheet sign" [Letter].** *JAMA.* 1984;251:891.

In despair, some patients with acquired immunodeficiency syndrome (AIDS) pull the hospital bedsheet up over their heads. Adams saw this frequently enough to regard it as a sign of AIDS-associated exogenous depression.

756. **Paauw DS, Wenrich MD, Curtis JR, et al. Ability of primary care physicians to recognize physical findings associated with HIV infection.** *JAMA.* 1995;274:1380-2.

Revealed a terrifying incompetence: despite a history provided by a standardized patient (patient instructor) directing attention toward a cutaneous Kaposi sarcoma or hairy leukoplakia of the mouth, the majority of the attending physicians studied did not even observe that there was any abnormal physical sign in the organ system in question at all, and half of those who saw that something was amiss could not diagnose the problem. The statistics with generalized lymphadenopathy were even more dismal.

757. **Schneiderman H, Garibaldi RA. Physical examination of HIV-infected patients (3-part article).** *Consultant.* 1990;30:33-8, 41-4, 47-8, 50-1, 55-6, 61-3.

A lengthy, three-part survey of a host of signs, principally those found in frank AIDS, but in some instances, those associated with earlier-stage HIV infection as well.

758. Cunha BA, Strampfer MJ. Clinical clues to AIDS: recognizing the dermatologic and nondermatologic manifestations. *Postgrad Med.* 1988;83:165-74, 177-9.

A survey describing signs of the condition, with several illustrations.

Skin, nails, hair

759. **Daniel CR, Norton A, Scher RK. The spectrum of nail disease in patients with human immunodeficiency virus infection.** *J Am Acad Derm.* **1992;27:93-7.**

Demonstrates that chalky white onychomycosis of fingernails suggests underlying HIV infection, as does dermatophytosis of all ten fingernails, the latter being more common when the T4 cell count falls below $100/mm^3$.

760. **Fallon T Jr, Abell E, Kingsley L, et al. Telangiectasias of the anterior chest in homosexual men.** *Ann Intern Med.* **1986;105:679-82.**

Color photographs illustrate a lesion significantly but not exclusively associated with HIV infection. Histologic study of lesions refines the association.

761. **Furth PA, Kazakis AM. Nail pigmentation changes associated with azidothymidine (zidovudine).** *Ann Intern Med.* **1987;107:350.**

The changes resemble those caused by some cancer chemotherapy agents.

762. **Koehler JE, LeBoit PE, Egbert BM, Berger TG. Cutaneous vascular lesions and disseminated cat-scratch disease in patients with the acquired immunodeficiency syndrome (AIDS) and AIDS-related complex.** *Ann Intern Med.* **1988;109:449-55.**

Shows that the purple-red skin nodules can be mistaken for Kaposi sarcoma. They fail to regress with therapy for that condition and respond dramatically to appropriate antimicrobials.

763. **Leonidas J-R. Hair alteration in black patients with the acquired immunodeficiency syndrome.** *Cutis.* **1987;39:537-8.**

Describes how curly capital (head) hair of black persons with AIDS can straighten spontaneously. The significance is unknown.

Eyes

764. **Bloom JN, Palestine AG. The diagnosis of cytomegalovirus retinitis.** *Ann Intern Med.* **1988;109:963-9.**

Splendid color photographs and a clear description of both cytomegalovirus and its major ophthalmoscopic differential diagnoses in the setting of AIDS.

765. deSmet MD. Differential diagnosis of retinitis and choroiditis in patients with acquired immunodeficiency syndrome. *Am J Med.* 1992;92(suppl 2A):17S-21S.

Well written, if highly specialized. The paper by Bloom and Palestine (reference 764) still remains the single most useful article on this topic.

766. deSmet MD, Nussenbatt RB. Ocular manifestations of AIDS. *JAMA.* 1991;266:3019-22.

A concise, practical review; clinically applicable.

767. Heinemann M-H. Characteristics of cytomegalovirus retinitis in patients with acquired immunodeficiency syndrome. *Am J Med.* 1992;92(suppl 2A):12S-16S.

Succinct, authoritative help in distinguishing this infection from cotton-wool spots and in getting a "first handle" on this common, devastating problem.

Mouth and face

768. Anonymous. Orofacial manifestations of HIV infection. *Lancet.* 1988; 1:976-7.

A brief listing and description of many common problems. HIV infection frequently produces signs that, when carefully looked for, can alert the dentist, otorhinolaryngologist, or internist to the diagnosis.

769. Bach MC, Valenti AJ, Howell DA, Smith TJ. Odynophagia from aphthous ulcers of the pharynx and esophagus in the acquired immunodeficiency syndrome (AIDS). *Ann Intern Med.* 1988;109:338-9.

Discusses how these lesions are easily mistaken for any of a plethora of infections. They can be effectively treated only if correctly diagnosed. Includes excellent illustrations.

770. Schulten EA, ten Kate RW, van der Waal I. The impact of oral examination on the Centers for Disease Control classification of subjects with human immunodeficiency virus infection. *Arch Intern Med.* 1990; 150:1259-61.

Demonstrates that, in a person believed to have asymptomatic seropositivity, findings such as thrush and oral Kaposi sarcoma often actually indicate overt AIDS.

771. Weinert M, Grimes RM, Lynch DP. Oral manifestations of HIV infection. *Ann Intern Med.* 1996;125:485-96.

Extensive catalogue with vivid illustrations. Apt discussion of the frequency of the 16 leading oral complications of HIV infection. Wonderful table describing the extremely probing 4-minute oral examination. A classic that will be widely used for a very long time.

772. Phelan JA, Saltzman BR, Friedland GH, Klein RS. Oral findings in patients with acquired immunodeficiency syndrome. *Oral Surg Oral Med Oral Pathol.* 1987;64:50-6.

Good older summary despite misplacement of photographs for illustrations 1 and 3 (each is captioned as the other).

Lymph nodes

773. **Abrams DI, Lewis BJ, Beckstead JH, et al. Persistent diffuse lymphaden-opathy in homosexual men: endpoint or prodrome?** *Ann Intern Med.* **1984;100:801-8.**

A very early description of lymphadenopathic AIDS-related complex in 70 men. Careful catalogue of the particular node groups involved. Does not answer the title question.

774. **Aguado JM, Castrillo JM. Lymphadenitis as a characteristic manifesta-tion of disseminated tuberculosis in intravenous drug abusers infected with human immunodeficiency virus.** *J Infect.* **1987;14:191-3.**

Discusses how in AIDS, infection with *Mycobacterium avium-intracellulare* complex is likely to affect deep but not peripheral nodes. Here, *M. tubercu-losis* produced superficial, palpable lymphadenopathy, hilar lymphadenopa-thy, or both, without other organ involvement.

775. **Malin A, Ternouth I, Sarbah S. Epitrochlear lymph nodes as marker of HIV disease in sub-Saharan Africa.** *BMJ.* **1994;309:1550-1.**

In a Zimbabwean hospital where more than half of unselected adults had antibody to HIV, palpable epitrochlear lymph nodes gave a positive predic-tive value of 85% for HIV infection.

Cardiorespiratory systems

776. **Bhat S, Heurich AE, Vaquer RA, et al. Hypertrophic osteoarthropathy associated with** *Pneumocystis carinii* **pneumonia in AIDS.** *Chest.* **1989; 96:1208-9.**

The extreme rarity of clubbing, let alone of full-blown hypertrophic osteo-arthropathy as described here, in even the most extraordinary pulmonary infections in AIDS, testifies to our primitive knowledge about both AIDS-associated lung disease and clubbing.

Limbs and locomotor system

777. **Abramson SB, Odajnyk CM, Grieco AJ, et al. Hyperalgesic pseudo-thrombophlebitis: new syndrome in male homosexuals.** *Am J Med.* **1985; 78:317-20.**

Discusses a new finding that so closely resembles venous thrombosis that it leads to phlebography in some instances. It is also readily confused with bac-terial cellulitis.

778. Davey RT Jr, Margolis D, Kleiner D, et al. Digital necrosis and disseminated *Pneumocystis carinii* infection after aerosolized pentamidine prophylaxis. *Ann Intern Med.* 1989;111:681-2.

Describes how extrapulmonary pneumocystosis occurs in this setting with particular frequency and virulence.

Anorectal and genital areas

779. Schneiderman H, Nzeako UC. Severe, recurrent perianal herpes lesions in HIV, and diverse anorectal disorders in AIDS. *Consultant.* 1996; 36:1243-7.

Describes what was an original index condition for HIV in the first cluster of articles in the *New England Journal of Medicine* (*see* reference 780), and is now a source of terrible discomfort rather than of diagnostic difficulty.

780. Siegal FP, Lopez C, Hammer GS, et al. Severe acquired immunodeficiency in male homosexuals, manifested by chronic perianal ulcerative herpes simplex lesions. *N Engl J Med.* 1981;305:1439-44.

The appalling severity, with ongoing necrosis, does not resemble any other familiar sexually transmitted condition. Nor is it like herpesvirus infection in any other kind of host except perhaps the organ-transplant recipient.

Neurologic and mental status

781. Jones BN, Teng EL, Folstein MF, Harrison KS. A new bedside test of cognition for patients with HIV infection. *Ann Intern Med.* 1993;119:1001-4.

Describes the Mental Alternations Test (MAT), a well-conceived screening instrument. Only attention and concentration are directly tested. As predictor of Folstein scores, it is probably good ($r = 0.68$). Appears to be an adequate screening for otherwise asymptomatic patients. Poor performance on this test constitutes reason to take the Mini-Mental State Examination. The premise that the latter is too lengthy for routine screening can be debated. However, serial assessment of brain function in AIDS patients is absolutely necessary because of the high incidence of HIV dementia and of dementing brain infections and neoplasm. If the MAT accomplishes this, it will have made a great mark notwithstanding its limited scope.

Other Patients with Special Needs

Adolescents and children

782. **Cope EB, Antony JH. Normal values for the two-point discrimination test.** *Pediatr Neurol.* **1992;8:251-4.**

According to the authors, 6-year-olds can cooperate satisfactorily with the test, which may be the first to disclose subtle sensory impairment. The most useful material in this article may be that concerning how to secure optimal interest, engagement, and meaningful results in any examination that requires cooperation from *any* patient who is less socialized and motivated than the usual healthy adult: application goes well beyond pediatrics.

783. **Galazka SS. Clinical magic and the art of examining children.** *J Fam Pract.* **1984;18:229-32.**

Several major behavioral suggestions apply in varying degree to adolescents, retarded adults, demented patients, psychotic patients, and others.

784. **Rapp CE Jr. The adolescent patient.** *Ann Intern Med.* **1983;99:52-60.**

Demonstrates that the objectives of the interview and examination of adolescents differ somewhat from those of adults, as do methods and even the doctor-patient relationship.

785. Yaffe ME. Rectal examination in adolescent males [Letter]. *Ann Intern Med.* 1983;99:574.

Thoughtful follow-up to the preceding article (reference 784): "For a teenage boy struggling with sexual identity, a genito-rectal examination . . . [can] precipitate homosexual panic." Careful explanation of purpose is needed, analogous to the first pelvic examination of a young girl.

Alcoholism

786. **Belton H. Lateral nystagmus: a specific diagnostic sign of ethyl alcohol intoxication.** *N Z Med J.* **1987;100:534-5.**

A police surgeon's correlation of blood levels with the presence of nystagmus on lateral gaze (not *extreme* lateral gaze, in which the finding is normal).

787. Clarren SK. Recognition of fetal alcohol syndrome. *JAMA.* 1981; 245:2436-9.

Classic paper, although not smooth-flowing. An astute and articulate description of the syndrome, vivid color photographs, and two very helpful tables.

788. Espinoza P, Ducot B, Pelletier G, et al. Interobserver agreement in the physical diagnosis of alcoholic liver disease. *Dig Dis Sci.* 1987;32:244-7.

Inter-rater reproducibility is limited, but the methods appear different from what constitutes routine clinical practice, and there is no reference standard. One cannot infer from where the data in Table 4, a key table, were derived.

789. Feussner JR, Linfors EW, Blessing CL, Starmer CF. Computed tomography brain scanning in alcohol withdrawal seizures: value of the neurologic examination. *Ann Intern Med.* 1981;94:519-22.

Unless such patients have had head trauma, no surgically correctable lesions are missed by omitting computed tomography when physical examination shows no focal neurologic deficits. Similar results apply with other neurologic symptoms in this population.

790. Rudzinski M, Stankaitis JA. Recognizing the alcoholic patient [Letter]. *N Engl J Med.* 1989;320:125-6.

Discusses how asking three simple questions at the time of any acute injury allow one to capitalize on a chance to identify the 10% of American adults with a drinking problem: "Was alcohol involved in the injury? Have you ever had a drinking problem? Have you consumed alcohol within the past 24 hours?"

Anorexia and bulimia

791. Schneiderman H, Eisenberg E. Bulimia: a dangerous variant of anorexia with oral physical signs. *Consultant.* 1995;35:1695-700.

Reviews the mechanism and appearance of perimylolysis, enamel erosion from exposure to acid vomitus that can yellow and erode the back surface of upper teeth as well as leave restorative metal material sticking out after the tooth around it has been rotted by acid.

792. Peterson DS, Barkmeier WW. Oral signs of frequent vomiting in anorexia. *Am Fam Physician.* 1983;27:199-200.

These signs, including the above and parotid enlargement, serve particularly well when the disorder includes denial of bulimic behavior. Can be used in adolescent screening.

Comatose and unresponsive patients

793. Henry JA, Woodruff GHA. A diagnostic sign in states of apparent unconsciousness. *Lancet.* **1978;2:920-1.**

If the eyes deviate equally downward whether the right lateral decubitus or the left lateral decubitus position has been assumed, voluntary control is operative. Thus, depending on the setting, either pseudocoma or pseudo-seizure may be diagnosed for the episode under observation. The authors are fully note that this does not prove that genuine seizures have not occurred at other times.

794. Noda S, Ito H, Umezaki H, Minato S. Hip flexion-abduction to elicit asterixis in unresponsive patients. *Ann Neurol.* **1985;18:96-7.**

An attempt to extend the spectrum of patients in whom one can obtain this valuable although nonspecific sign. Unfortunately, the sign cannot be produced at all in true coma, when it might be the most helpful in pointing to a metabolic rather than a structural cause.

Critical care unit patients (critically ill persons)

795. Baldwin JG Jr. The healing touch [Editorial]. *Am J Med.* **1986;80:1.**

A personal reflection emphasizes how physician contact helps patients in ways that high technology cannot supplant. Incidentally reveals what is most in jeopardy of being forgotten in the critical care setting.

796. Dobb GJ, Coombs LJ. Clinical examination of patients in the intensive care unit. *Br J Hosp Med.* **1987;38:102-8.**

One of the very few published treatments of this vital topic.

797. McNally D. The technique of physical examination in the ICU: how data gleaned in 30 seconds improves 'high-tech' care. *J Crit Illness.* **1990; 5:1305-12.**

Describes a rapid series of questions, thoughts, and movements of the palpating hand, the inspecting eye, and the ausculting ear that enable the examiner to categorize sudden, calamitous change in a critical care unit patient.

798. Pierson JC, Lawlor KB, Steck WD. Pen push purpura: iatrogenic nail bed hemorrhages in the intensive care unit. *Cutis.* **1993;51:422-3.**

Case report of little hematomas at the lunulae that resulted from attempts to demonstrate pain sensibility in a comatose patient by pressing with a pen.

799. **Shelly MP, Church JJ. Bowel sounds during intermittent positive pressure ventilation [Letter].** *Anaesthesia.* **1987;42:207-9.**

Discusses how patients on mechanical ventilation, especially if therapeutically paralyzed, might not swallow air. An absence of bowel sounds in these patients therefore does *not* mean an ileus is present.

Deaf and hearing-impaired persons

800. **Lotke M. She won't look at me.** *Ann Intern Med.* **1995;123:54-7.**

Potent plea for measures that ease the medical interface for hearing-impaired patients. Much practical advice. Strong advocacy for certified American Sign Language (ASL) interpreters. Lip reading is unsatisfactory. Treats ASL as a language entirely different from written English, with implications that are not obvious to the "outsider."

801. **Reisman G, Scanlan J, Kemp K. Medical interpreting for hearing-impaired patients.** *JAMA.* **1977;237:2397-8.**

Asserts that family members of the hearing-impaired patient should not serve as medical interpreters and that note writing is often inappropriate. Simple but not obvious guidelines.

Demented and retarded persons

802. **Benesch CG, McDaniel KD, Cox C, Hamill RW. End-stage Alzheimer's disease: Glasgow coma scale and the neurologic examination.** *Arch Neurol.* **1993;50:1309-15.**

In the final phases of degenerative dementia, due to a floor effect, the Mini-Mental State Examination does not characterize further loss of function. Myoclonus becomes more frequent, and so do dyskinesias, even without neuroleptic use. The Glasgow scale, although developed for an entirely different clinical problem, offers some discriminant value.

803. **Burns A, Jacoby R, Levy R. Neurological signs in Alzheimer's disease.** *Age Ageing.* **1991;20:45-51.**

Rigorous correlation with computed axial tomography and standardized cognitive tests. The most striking finding may be the 5% prevalence of myoclonus, which is so often adduced to raise suspicion that the illness is Creutzfeldt-Jakob disease.

804. Drews RC. Mirror fixation. *Am J Ophthalmol.* **1976;82:938-9.**

Describes a method to simplify funduscopy in the inattentive or incapable: having the patient stare at his or her own reflection in a mirror kept within the visual field.

805. Freeman BJ, Roy RR, Hemmick S. Extinction of a phobia of physical examination in a seven-year-old mentally retarded boy: a case study. *Behav Res Ther.* **1976;14:63-4.**

Psychologically sensitive statements on overcoming a problem that is not limited to children or retarded persons.

806. Molloy DW, Clarnette RM, McIlroy WE, et al. Clinical significance of primitive reflexes in Alzheimer's disease. *J Am Geriatr Soc.* **1991; 39:1160-3.**

In this study, cognition appeared not to be significantly different among patients with Alzheimer disease who had snout, suck, grasp, or palmomental reflexes compared with those who did not. Nevertheless, the patients with primitive reflexes had more rigidity and more behavioral dyscontrol.

807. Schneiderman H. Flexion contractures and the physical examination of patients with advanced dementia. *Consultant.* **1993;33:93-4, 98.**

Examinations of skin, mouth, abdomen, perineum, and joints may have the highest yield for quality of life in such patients.

808. Walstra GJM, van Gool WA. The need for a "second witness" in diagnosing dementia. *J Am Geriatr Soc.* **1995;43:1176-7.**

Discusses problems with families that may minimize or exaggerate cognitive loss, either because the family lacks insight about the patient's problem or because the family seeks to control the outcome of the medical visit. The family as collateral informant (source of collateral history) is not always reliable.

Difficult and hostile persons

809. Groves JE. Taking care of the hateful patient. *N Engl J Med.* **1978; 298:883-7.**

A supremely insightful and helpful article for all clinicians, detailing four groups of patients that induce negative feelings in the physician, feelings that are to be used for clinical insight about the patient and not merely quashed: dependent clingers who breed aversion; entitled demanders who evoke a wish to counterattack; manipulative help-rejecters who make the physician depressed and self-doubting; and self-destructive deniers who inspire malicious thoughts.

Disabled (physically challenged) persons

810. Peters L. Women's health care: approaches in delivery to physically disabled women. *Nurse Pract.* 1982;7:34, 36-7, 48.

Discusses attitudinal requirements, equipment, techniques, and patience. Applicable to generalists, internists, and gynecologists.

Drug abusers

811. Babenco HD, Roche J, Schneiderman H. Talc emboli of the retinal vessels in an intravenous drug abuser: a vivid ophthalmoscopic finding. *Consultant.* 1994;34:231-2.

Describes this unique finding, which one might envision as prevented by the pulmonary capillary filter.

812. Cherubin CE, Sapira JD. The medical complications of drug addiction and the medical assessment of the intravenous drug user: 25 years later. *Ann Intern Med.* 1993;119:1017-28.

Less explicit about individual interview and examination findings than the same authors' earlier treatments of the subject, but nevertheless powerful and useful. The length of the catalogue of street names of drugs is exceeded only by that of the medical complications of abuse.

813. Sapira JD. The narcotic addict as a medical patient. *Am J Med.* 1968;45:555-88.

An old classic, still very much worth reading even though the drugs of abuse, routes of administration, and associated disorders have changed considerably.

814. Larkin RF. The callus of crack cocaine [Letter]. *N Engl J Med.* 1990;323:685.

Shows that such calluses result from endless manipulation of the serrated wheel of a butane lighter. Still another illustration of the variety and sadness of addicts' lesions.

815. Schneiderman H, Eisenberg E, Krutchkoff DJ. Cocaine dental erosions and other physical findings in cocaine users. *Consultant.* 1994;34:545-6.

Describes features in the mouth, vital signs, skin, heart and lungs, and neurologic examination.

816. Krutchkoff DJ, Eisenberg E, O'Brien JE, Ponzillo JJ. Cocaine-induced dental erosions [Letter]. *N Engl J Med.* 1990;322:408.

The acid produced when cocaine mixes with saliva erodes teeth and gums in a striking fashion, as illustrated vividly in an accompanying photograph.

817. Tennant F. The rapid eye test to detect drug abuse. *Postgrad Med.* 1988; 84:108-14.

Describes simple maneuvers to detect ocular abnormalities indicative of recent substance use. The test is claimed to have good sensitivity and specificity whenever two or more "primary findings" (ptosis, abnormal pupillary size or reactivity, nystagmus, nonconvergence) are present. No data are presented to substantiate the claim.

818. Zamora-Quezada JC, Dinerman H, Stadecker MG, Kelly JJ. Muscle and skin infarction after free-basing cocaine (crack). *Ann Intern Med.* 1988;108:564-5.

Describes prominent physical findings, illustrated in color, along with highly abnormal laboratory results.

819. Zorc TG, O'Donnell AE, Holt RW, et al. Bilateral pyopneumothorax secondary to intravenous drug abuse. *Chest.* 1988;93:645-7.

Color photograph vividly illustrates the supraclavicular puncture marks that accompany "shooting the pocket" in intravenous drug abuse. Detection of these should prompt a search for pleuropulmonary complications.

Homeless persons

820. Schneiderman H. Frostbite, health needs, and physical examination of homeless persons. *Consultant.* 1994;34:1577-83.

Emphasizes examination of the feet and skin, and assessment of nutrition, hydration, and mental state.

Homosexual patients

821. Owen WF Jr. The clinical approach to the male homosexual patient. *Med Clin North Am.* 1986;70:499-535.

The guidelines are rich not only in specifics but also in common sense and sensitivity. Adherence to these insights can help one avoid hurting the substantial fraction of all patients who do not confide sexual preference to their physicians.

Immigrants, non-English speakers, and differing cultural expectations

822. Ebden P, Bhatt A, Carey OJ, Harrison B. The bilingual consultation. *Lancet.* 1988;1:347.

Taped interviews of an English-speaking physician, bilingual interpreter, and Gujarati-speaking patient. Review of translated transcripts revealed severely misleading statements that occurred for both cultural and linguistic reasons and would have prevented correct diagnosis.

823. Ghoda MK. Bilingual consultation [Letter]. *Lancet.* 1988;1:648.

Striking statements; for example, that foreign graduates must learn five English alternatives for "backside," yet the Royal Colleges have no place for cross-cultural (or transcultural, as it is now also called) communication in their curricula.

824. Hostetter MK, Johnson D. Medical examination of the internationally adopted child: screening for infectious diseases and developmental delay. *Postgrad Med.* 1996;99:70-82.

Although most of the focus is on laboratory evaluation, the basic history is vital: the specific issues vary with country of origin, and not only with disease prevalence there.

825. Qureshi B. How to avoid pitfalls in ethnic medical history, examination, and diagnosis [Editorial]. *J R Soc Med.* 1992;85:65-6.

Valid points include the need for a link-person who translates culture as well as language. Different descriptions of pain, senses of privacy around age and religion, and issues about the role of touching in the clinical interaction. Also discusses the taboo nature of the anogenital examination in Eastern culture. Important caveats for every physician to study.

826. Barone TL, Bhakta P, Jayanthi V, Mayberry J. Examination of the breast in minority groups. *Surg Gynecol Obstet.* 1992;174:325.

Ill-titled: the intended patient population is people of little education or with cultural resistance to breast exposure for the physician. Well-meaning but misguided demonstration of texture by having the patient practice on the closed eyelid over the globe, thereby minimizing exposure of the breast (*see* Qureshi's article, reference 825). To use the development of fixation as a trigger to seek examination is to wait until it is too late in the natural history of breast cancer.

827. Schneiderman H. Coin-rubbing, folk remedies, and physical examination of immigrants. *Consultant.* 1995;35:1349-52.

Illustrations and limited but perhaps surprising text.

Malingerers, hysterics, and extreme symptom-amplifiers

828. Keane JR. Hysterical gait disorders: 60 cases. *Neurology.* 1989;39:586-9.

Discusses the recognition of and therapy for these disorders. Shows that sophisticated imaging is not needed if the clinician has the mindset and experience to be suspicious. The value of assessing gait as the best single test of neurologic function is also restated.

829. **Keane JR. Neuro-ophthalmic signs and symptoms of hysteria.** *Neurology.* **1982;32:757-62.**

Physiologic sophistication highlights case histories that show how to uncover voluntary, abnormal physical signs, some devilishly clever.

830. **Keane JR. Wrong-way deviation of the tongue with hysterical hemiparesis.** *Neurology.* **1986;36:1406-7.**

Discusses how the malingerer may deviate the tongue *away* from the side of a simulated hemiparesis, something that occurs only with the rarest of medullary strokes. A wonderful clue in an area where we all need help, from the established master of the domain.

831. **Murray HW, Tuazon CU, Guerrero IC, et al. Urinary temperature: a clue to early diagnosis of factitious fever.** *N Engl J Med.* **1977;296:23-4.**

Fine science does not depend on fancy equipment. Use of their nomogram can truncate needless work-up.

832. **Tager RM. Simulated disability.** *J Occup Med.* **1985;27:915-6.**

Behavioral features, characteristics of language (for example, overly medical and legal) and history, and examination features that help one spot fakes. Suitable warnings about the difference between malingering and the common phenomenon of "benign symptom exaggeration."

Mentally ill persons

833. **Dahlquist LM, Gil KM, Kalfus GR, et al. Enhancing an autistic girl's cooperation with gynecological examinations.** *Clin Pediatr.* **1984;23:203.**

Psychologists and pediatricians formed an intricate but rapid and effective plan, transferable to any part of the examination and to any patient with disabling examination phobia or limited comprehension.

Neutropenic patients, cancer therapy patients, and bone marrow transplant recipients

834. **Carl W. Oral manifestations of systemic chemotherapy and their management.** *Semin Surg Oncol.* **1986;2:187-99.**

Authoritative, well-illustrated, and highly comprehensible information on the plethora of infectious and noninfectious problems to which the bone-marrow transplant recipient and other chemotherapy patients are subject.

835. **Gaspari AA, Lotze MT, Rosenberg SA, et al. Dermatologic changes associated with interleukin 2 administration.** *JAMA.* **1987;258:1624-9.**

Discusses common complications of a relatively new cancer therapy. These changes need to be recognized if they are to be treated optimally, without wasting the patient's time and money on exclusion of unrealistic alternatives.

836. **Schneiderman H, Tutschka PJ, Eisenberg E. Oral candidal infection and graft-versus-host disease in a bone marrow transplant recipient.** *Consultant.* **1996;36:517-24.**

Heavily illustrated. Combines insights of multiple disciplines.

837. Kolbinson DA, Schubert MM, Flournoy N, Truelove EL. Early oral changes following bone marrow transplantation. *Oral Surg Oral Med Oral Pathol.* 1988;66:130-8.

Discusses the wide variety of color changes and other alterations that occur after bone marrow transplantation, some reflecting treatable oral infectious complications.

838. **Sickles EA, Greene WH, Wiernik PH. Clinical presentation of infection in granulocytopenic patients.** *Arch Intern Med.* **1975;135:715-9.**

Frequency of specific signs and symptoms in the presence of carefully defined infection at one of five named sites. Fever, local erythema, and tenderness remained sensitive indicators when others were lost.

Obese patients

839. **Buchan NG. Breast examination in obese patients [Letter].** *Lancet.* **1976; 1:48.**

Discusses how the compression of pectoralis major renders interpectoral lymph nodes more accessible.

840. **Maxwell MH, Schroth PC, Waks AU, et al. Error in blood-pressure measurement due to incorrect cuff size in obese patients.** *Lancet.* **1982;2:33-6.**

Concerns overestimation with cuffs that are too small for thick arms and may cause erroneous diagnosis of hypertension in overweight patients. Derives correction formulae. Disputes then-standard American Heart Association guidelines.

Pregnant women and infertile couples

841. **Bauman JE. Basal body temperature: unreliable method of ovulation detection.** *Fertil Steril.* **1981;36:729-33.**

Demonstrates that this vital sign cannot be stretched to predict or record ovulation in any person.

842. Pirie AM, Quinn M. Vascular sounds in hypertensive pregnancy [Letter]. *Lancet.* **1996;347:618-9.**

Complex material about Korotkoff sounds IV and V, the upshot of which is that automated blood pressure measurements may miss proteinuric, pre-eclamptic hypertension of pregnancy.

Rape, assault, and torture victims

843. Cathcart LM, Berger P, Knazan B. Medical examination of torture victims applying for refugee status. *Can Med Assoc J.* **1979;121:179-80, 183-4.**

Discusses how medical evidence can make a major difference in granting of refugee status. Great patience, gentleness, and much time are needed to overcome a victim's terror and elicit the full story. Documentation is vital.

844. Hampton HL. Care of the woman who has been raped. *N Engl J Med.* **1995;332:234-7.**

Lucid, practical, compassionate, and professional treatment of a most painful topic. The focus is appropriately psychological as well as physical, legal as well as medical. Mentions date rape, battered wife syndrome, and the rape of women older than 50 years (60,000 rapes occurring per year in this age group in the United States): Rape victims can be seen by any physician. Besides the need to assess the genitalia, anus, and mouth, one must look elsewhere for lacerations, which may represent stab wounds. An essential article.

845. Wertheimer AJ. Examination of the rape victim. *Postgrad Med.* 1982;71:173-6, 179-80.
Older but worthwhile treatment, with sound mixture of medical, legal, and humane aspects.

846. Levitt CJ. Medical evaluation of the sexually abused child. *Prim Care.* **1993;20:343-54.**

Much material on the taking and interpretation of the history. The section, "A caring approach to examining children," is well named. Illustrations and discussion, among other issues, of hymenal lesions that are innocuous versus those caused by abuse.

847. Hobbs CJ, Wynne JM. Examination findings in legally confirmed child sexual abuse: it's normal to be normal [Letter]. *Pediatrics.* 1996;47:148-50.
Striking disagreement with other authorities on the significance of several basic findings and on the interpretation of colposcopic photographs of the anogenital region. Expected consensus in this area does not yet exist.

848. Schneiderman H. The mark of a survivor of the Nazi concentration camps. *Consultant.* **1992;32:83-4.**

Mention of the number-and-letter tattoos placed on human beings in these sites of torture. Brief discussion of the recognition and treatment of Holocaust survivors, and of the absence of a comparable physical sign by which to know others who have lived through hell.

Renal disease: patients with endstage renal failure

849. **Anonymous. Diastolic murmurs in renal failure [Leading Article]. *Lancet*. 1986;1:482.**

Discusses how these murmurs often represent functional semilunar valve insufficiency. They frequently abate with correction of hypervolemia-associated systemic or pulmonary arterial hypertension.

850. **Callen JP. Cutaneous nephrology. In: Callen JP, Jorizzo JL, Greer KE, et al, eds. *Dermatological Signs of Internal Disease*. 2nd ed. Philadelphia: WB Saunders; 1995:307-11.**

Discusses the cutaneous complications of uremia and the markers of some of its causes. See reference 175 for full citation of the book.

851. **Klaasen-Broekema N, van Bijsterveld OP. Red eyes in renal failure. *Br J Ophthalmol*. 1992;76:268-71.**

Two patterns are discerned: one that is localized and adjoins calcium deposits in the cornea and conjunctiva, mimicking inflammation of a pinguecula; the other that is more diffuse and relates to extreme elevation of the serum calcium level.

852. **Rault R. Transmitted murmurs in patients undergoing hemodialysis. *Arch Intern Med*. 1989;149:1392-3.**

Discusses how patients on hemodialysis often have transmitted bruits to the cervical, supraclavicular, and infraclavicular areas. Identification of these transmitted sounds by their disappearance upon very cautious, momentary compression of the fistula may avoid costly diagnostic work-up.

853. **Wheeler SD. Long-term hemodialysis and supraclavicular bruits: a method of examination. *JAMA*. 1982;247:1026.**

Describes how brief, gentle occlusion of the arterial flow proximal to the dialysis fistula obliterates a bruit only when it arises from the fistula.

Reserved, depressed, and withdrawn patients

854. **Havens LL. Taking a history from the difficult patient. *Lancet*. 1978; 1:138-40.**

Discusses how fear, repression, and concealment cloud responses. Internists can use strategies for minimizing this obstruction as effectively as do psychiatrists.

855. Rohde P. The withdrawn patient. *Practitioner.* **1978;220:223-7.**

Friendly tone and many case histories. Helps one to recognize withdrawn patients, to identify an organic or psychological cause, and to get a proper history from the patient or informant. Includes mental status examination and differential diagnosis.

Case Presentation

856. Bennett HJ. How to survive a case presentation. *Chest*. 1985;88:292-4.

A helpfully humorous treatment of an important topic by the leading physician-teacher-humorist.

857. Billings JA, Stoeckle JD. Oral case presentations. In: Billings JA, Stoeckle JD, eds. *The Clinical Encounter*. Chicago: Year Book; 1989:259-69.

Distinctive comments on what is needed and useful in several variations of oral information transfer between health professionals. Particularly clear on the differences between written and spoken case summaries.

858. Kroenke K. The case presentation: stumbling blocks and stepping stones. *Am J Med*. 1985;79:605-8.

Discusses how to transmit information in a format "neither soporific nor skimpy." Excellent, detailed advice. The article itself is a model of lucidity.

859. Vaughan SC. Joint authorship in the physician-patient interaction. *Pharos*. 1990;53:38-42.

An insightful examination of the change from first-person voice to objectification in the interpretation of the patient's narrative. Pertinent to case presentation, to history taking in general, and to the creation of write-ups.

860. Yurchak PM. A guide to medical case presentations. *Res Staff Phys*. 1981;27:109-11, 114-5.

Beautifully organized, clearly stated, concise, and useful remarks on how to transmit the results of a work-up effectively.

Teaching Bedside Skills

861. Benbassat J, Meroz N. The foam sponge as a teaching aid in the examination of the chest. *Med Educ.* **1988;22:554-5.**

Describes a simulator of the pulmonary parenchyma's poor sound transmission.

862. Block MR, Coulehan JL. Teaching the difficult interview in a required course on medical interviewing. *J Med Educ.* **1987;62:35-40.**

Excellent means of clearing the barriers to acquisition of medical data, by two authors whose textbook on history taking also merits attention.

863. Grady MJ, Earll JM. Teaching physical diagnosis in the nursing home. *Am J Med.* **1990;88:519-21.**

Discusses a way around the problems of using hospital inpatients (too sick, too many investigations, endless interruptions). As with any other endeavor, success will be proportionate to the effort expended in organization and execution.

864. Fitzgerald FT. Bedside teaching. *West J Med.* **1993;158:418-20.**

Astute discussion of the need to get to the bedside on teaching rounds, the psychic barriers on the part of faculty and housestaff who fear humiliating public exposure of their imperfections, and the remedies for these problems.

865. Hamburger S, Guthrie D, Smith PG, Shaffer K. Teaching the pelvic examination in an internal medicine residency program. *West J Med.* **1981;134:547-8.**

Several useful insights about patient-instructors.

866. Lipkin M Jr, Quill TE, Napodano RJ. The medical interview: a core curriculum for residencies in internal medicine. *Ann Intern Med.* **1984; 100:277-84.**

The much expanded sense of the term "medical interview" used here leads to a formidable, desirable curriculum.

867. **Mangione S, Nieman LZ, Gracely E, Kaye D. The teaching and practice of cardiac auscultation during internal medicine and cardiology training: a nationwide survey.** *Ann Intern Med.* **1993;119:47-54.**

Alarming study uncovering the absence of structured teaching of auscultation in the United States, and the expected ramifications thereof—namely, ineffective auscultators.

868. St. Clair EW, Oddone EZ, Waugh RA, et al. Assessing housestaff diagnostic skills using a cardiology patient simulator. *Ann Intern Med.* 1992;117:751-6.

Discusses how housestaff in a prestigious training program performed dismally in identifying mitral regurgitation as well as some tougher murmurs.

869. **Marsden PD. Semiologia.** *BMJ.* **1991;302:645-6.**

Inspirational account of teaching rounds.

870. **Mayo-Smith MF, Gordon V, Gillie E, Brett A. Teaching physical diagnosis in the nursing home: a prospective, controlled trial.** *J Am Geriatr Soc.* **1991;39:1085-8.**

As described by these authors, medical students like the site but find cognitively impaired patients frustrating for history-taking. Among the advantages are fewer interruptions, less noise, and a high prevalence of abnormal physical findings.

871. **Reuler JB, Nardone DA, Elliot DL, Girard DE. Education for clinical medicine: an annotated bibliography of recent literature.** *Ann Intern Med.* **1982;97:624-9.**

Encompasses a different range of topics than the present bibliography, and includes excellent choices on instruction and competence in bedside examination. Although the citations are no longer recent literature, they still afford valuable insights.

872. **Robinson JK, McGaghie WC. Skin cancer detection in a clinical practice examination with standardized patients.** *J Am Acad Dermatol.* **1996;34:709-11.**

In this report, patient-instructors had an 8-mm pseudo-melanoma applied by cosmetics! Only one of 285 senior medical students spotted this although it was strategically placed for optimum noticeability during history-taking and other cues were available. Implications about missing easily recognized lesions while they remain in a window of curability are dreadful.

873. Schneiderman H. The morgue: a neglected classroom for physical diagnosis. *Conn Med.* 1983;47:8-12.

Describes how to hone inspection, palpation, and percussion skills by practice just before autopsy dissection, with immediate correlation.

874. Wallis LA, Tardiff K, Deane K, Frings J. Teaching associates and the male genitorectal exam. *J Am Med Wom Assoc.* 1984;39:57-8, 62.

Still more patient-instructors, highly trained to provide not only their own anatomic parts but also informed and sentient feedback.

Author Index

Bauer MS, 222
Baughman RP, 328
Baum J, 219
Bauman JE, 841
Baumann MH, 316
Beatty RM, 665
Beaven DW, 199
Beck IT, 464
Beck L, 223
Beck LH, 677
Becker WG, 717
Beckstead JH, 773
Beder S, 200
Beede SD, 441
Beek WC, 732
Beitman RG, 264
Bellantonio S, 738
Bellet PS, 51
Belmin J, 127
Belmont L, 301
Belton H, 786
Benbadis SR, 265
Benbassat J, 861
Benchimol A, 378
Benesch CG, 802
Bengmark S, 469
Benjamin S, 668
Benjamin SB, 480
Bennett DH, 470
Bennett HJ, 856
Benson RC Jr, 553
Berger P, 843
Berger SR, 131
Berger TG, 762
Bergman A, 584
Berk SL, 93, 506
Bernhard JD, 166, 195
Bernhardt DT, 588
Bess FH, 726
Betti R, 296
Betts T, 687
Bhakta P, 826
Bhat S, 776
Bhatt A, 822
Bickers DR, 182
Bickley LS, 44
Bicknell JM, 669
Bijsterveld OP van, 851

Billings JA, 857
Birge SJ, 697
Bismuth H, 179
Black FW, 695
Blank SG, 128
Blau JN, 52, 651
Blein BEK, 238
Blessing CL, 789
Bloch H, 21
Block MR, 862
Bloom JN, 764
Blower PW, 594
Blunt BA, 229
Blunt S, 684
Bole GG, 204
Bonerandi JJ, 184
Bono DP de, 46
Bosser SK, 514
Bouchard AG, 442
Bouffler LE, 626
Bouter LM, 600
Bouthillier D, 725
Bower JD, 201
Bowsher D, 641
Boyce JA, 166
Brady HR, 612
Brady PM, 245
Braekhus A, 731
Branch WT, 53
Brannon WL, 672
Braunstein GD, 307
Braverman IM, 174
Brearley S, 445
Brentnall E, 254
Breslin DJ, 624
Brett A, 870
Briggs RS, 722
Brik A, 423
Broadmore J, 559
Brocklehurst JC, 703
Brook G, 423
Brooks SE, 199
Brown C, 618
Brown JB, 54, 55, 56
Brown KL, 411
Brown RA, 742, 743
Brugada P, 353
Bruno A, 233

Brust JC, 681
Buchan NG, 839
Buchanan RG, 706
Buchsbaum DG, 706
Buckman R, 57
Bugge PM, 96
Bull DA, 234
Bunker CB, 190
Burch GE, 389
Burge DM, 554
Burket MW, 421
Burns A, 803
Bush I, 541
Butman SM, 403
Byrd BF, 290

C

Calin A, 35
Callaham M, 661
Callahan CW Jr, 496
Callen JP, 175, 176, 850
Campbell JA, 641
Campbell WB, 470
Camus M, 509, 510
Canfield DC, 365
Capel LH, 330, 331
Capellan J, 89
Caplan LR, 639, 685
Caputo GM, 619
Caranasos GJ, 740
Carbillet JP, 616
Carey OJ, 822
Carl W, 834
Carmel R, 183
Carpenter JL, 18
Carr-Gregg M, 559
Carson L, 36
Carter F, 36
Carter SS, 490
Cassell EJ, 58
Cassileth BR, 167
Castell DO, 480
Castle SC, 114
Castrillo JM, 774
Catalona WJ, 543
Cathcart LM, 843

Dumesic DA, 752
Dunnick NR, 493
Dupond JL, 616
Durkan JA, 628
Duroziez, 401
Dutton JL, 462
Dyck P, 595, 667

E

Earil JM, 863
Earis J, 322
Earis JE, 329
Earnest DL, 220
East of Ireland, Faculty, 116
Eastwood HD, 722
Eaton D, 108
Ebara S, 670
Ebden P, 822
Eckardt VF, 520
Egbert BM, 762
Ehrenkranz JR, 115
Eilen SD, 355
Einterz EM, 69
Eipper DF, 491
Eisen AZ, 160
Eisenberg E, 255, 268, 791, 815, 836
Elias PM, 191
Ellenby MI, 243
Elliot DL, 871
Elliott BG, 629
Ellis DL, 177
Elta G, 533
Elton RA, 518, 519
Ende J, 74, 499
Engedahl K, 731
Epstein O, 46
Espinoza P, 788
Eton D, 243
Etzel RA, 345
Everitt DE, 87
Ewy GA, 403, 453, 454

F

Faculty, East of Ireland, 116
Fairbank JCT, 597
Fallon T Jr, 760
Falstie-Jensen N, 446
Fante RG, 234
Fariselli G, 297
Farnett LE, 346
Farrior JB III, 631
Faryna A, 64
Fauver HE, 552
Feagan B, 433
Feingold KR, 191
Feinstein AR, 713
Feldberg MAM, 479
Feldman LJ, 261
Feldon SE, 221
Ferguson J, 380
Fernandez A, 125
Ferrucci L, 736, 737
Feussner JR, 482, 789
Fielding JF, 484-487
Fieselman JF, 150
Filler SJ, 274
Filly RA, 37
Finsterbush A, 610
Fiorini A, 192
Fisher EW, 247
Fisher ME, 198
Fisher TD, 85
Fitzgerald FT, 1, 38, 95, 864
Fitzpatrick TB, 160, 161, 168
Flack J, 134
Flanders WD, 345
Fletcher RH, 292
Fletcher SW, 292
Flickinger AL, 421
Flynn MD, 745
Foley AE, 633
Folland ED, 379
Folstein MF, 781
Forgacs P, 323
Forker AD, 39

Formas ME, 222
Formolo J, 20, 22
Forrester JS, 416
Forsell G, 387
Fortuin NJ, 397
Foster JH, 549
Fowler FD, 665
Fowler J, 36
Fowler NO, 143, 377, 425
Fox RA, 749
Frame PS, 4
Francis DM, 475
Frank CW, 2
Frank SH, 3
Frankl U, 610
Franklin C, 100
Franks PJ, 521, 523, 524
Fraser AG, 391
Fred HL, 237
Freeman BJ, 805
Freundlich JH, 446
Fried M, 196
Friedland GH, 772
Friedland JA, 19
Friedman GD, 525, 535, 539
Friedman IH, 256
Friedman M, 418
Friedman RJ, 169, 170
Friedman-Kien AE, 188
Frier BM, 437
Fries JF, 35
Frings J, 874
Frost HM, 613
Frost SS, 264
Fuji T, 670
Fuller B, 110
Fuller GN, 497
Fulop G, 694
Funahashi A, 338, 340
Furth PA, 761

G

Galazka SS, 783
Gallegos NC, 488

Hendriksen C, 96
Hendryx MS, 150
Henkind P, 227
Hennigan TW, 521, 523, 524
Henry JA, 615, 793
Hepper NG, 723
Herrinton LJ, 525
Herzog A, 61
Hess SP, 103
Heurich AE, 776
Hiatt RA, 539
Hill, 401
Hill JL, 698
Hill NS, 419
Hirakawa S, 406
Hitchcock ER, 655
Hitchings RA, 218
Hjalmarson A, 146
Hobbs CJ, 847
Hobsley M, 488
Hocken DB, 521, 524
Hodges M, 376
Hoekelman RA, 44
Hoffbrand BI, 84, 129
Holbrook JH, 12
Holford SK, 311
Holleman DR, 336
Holleman DR Jr, 342
Hollerbach AD, 148
Holt RW, 819
Holzberg M, 203
Hooper EM, 67
Hooper PL, 67
Hopkins LC, 277
Hoppenfeld S, 590
Horan DB, 548
Horan MA, 749
Horne D, 556
Hostetter MK, 824
Howard R, 710
Howard RJ, 97
Howe D, 208
Howell DA, 769
Howell JM, 117
Howell TH, 721
Humbert P, 616
Hunder GG, 592, 723

Hunt DK, 335
Hunter GC, 234
Hunter PA, 218
Hurley CM, 118
Hurst JW, 48, 220, 277, 348, 638
Huson S, 223
Hutton JD, 559

I

Ike RW, 608
Impallomeni M, 745
Insall RL, 447
Isaacs B, 714
Ishii T, 246
Ishmail AA, 380
Israel R, 740
Ito H, 794

J

Jacobsen BA, 446
Jacobson JS, 572
Jacoby R, 692, 803
Jahnigen DW, 728
James EM, 441
Jansen GT, 548
Jansen RWMM, 130
Jayanthi V, 826
Jenkyn LR, 658
Jensen AM, 96
Jensen JL, 263
Jewell L, 275
Johnson BE, 269
Johnson D, 824
Johnson DC, 343
Johnson FL, 621
Johnson GK, 64
Johnson JE, 18
Johnson JJ, 158
Johnston D, 30
Jolin SW, 117
Jonasson R, 387
Jones A, 124
Jones BN, 781

Jones D, 223
Jones FL Jr, 318
Jones N, 30
Jones WL, 233
Jorizzo JL, 175

K

Kadri N, 360
Kafka SP, 177
Kagan A, 206
Kahanovich S, 196
Kaisla T, 332
Kaleida PH, 250
Kalfus GR, 833
Kamal A, 703
Kampmeier RH, 7, 8
Kanski JJ, 216
Kantrowitz FG, 637
Kanzler G, 520
Kao K-P, 640
Kapila R, 90
Kaplan AI, 98
Kaplan MC, 408
Kar PM, 422
Karnegis JN, 360
Karr MD, 24
Kassirer JP, 62
Kate RW ten, 770
Katz GA, 634
Katz JN, 596, 635
Kaye D, 867
Kazakis AM, 761
Keane JR, 828-830
Keene M, 249
Keipper VL, 210
Kelly J, 818
Kelly JW, 171
Kemp K, 801
Kemple T, 522
Kenik JG, 204
Kenna C, 278
Kennedy GT, 138
Kenny RA, 142, 745
Keogh JAB, 492
Kerigan AT, 396
Kern DG, 337, 339

Lusk EJ, 167
Luutonen S, 141
Lynch DP, 771

M

MacFarlane IA, 641
Mackenzie TB, 70
Mackowiak PA, 119
Macleod DAD, 518
Mader SL, 140
Mador MJ, 153
Magalotti D, 507
Maganias NH, 224
Magee J, 562
Magee TR, 448
Mahowald ML, 623
Maisel AS, 370
Majerovitz SD, 709
Maleki-Yazdi R, 151
Maletta G, 733
Malin A, 775
Maloney MJ, 51
Mangione S, 867
Mann G, 610
Mann LC, 293
Mannino DM, 345
Manutsathit S, 688
Maranhao V, 371
Marantz PR, 408, 409
Marcus RH, 455
Mardsen PD, 869
Margolis D, 778
Margolis KL, 240
Margouleff D, 420
Maricq HR, 204
Markiewicz W, 423
Marsh K, 329
Martin L, 99
Martinez H, 404
Martyn CN, 437
Mashberg A, 260, 261
Maslin K, 225
Massey EW, 648, 672, 675
Masters AP, 420
Masuda S, 246

Matchar DB, 643
Mathews WC, 319, 513
Mathias S, 714
Maurice WL, 77
Maxwell MH, 840
Mayberry J, 826
Mayo-Smith MF, 870
McAllister K, 632
McBrien DJ, 436
McCaffree DR, 417
McCarty DJ, 666
McCombe PF, 597
McCormack DG, 31
McCullagh GC, 591
McCullough JA, 601
McCullough LB, 83
McDaniel KD, 802
McDermott J, 299
McDonnell M, 533
McElligott G, 302
McElwain TJ, 86
McFadden JP, 722
McGaghie WC, 872
McGee SR, 25
McGinnis LS, 305
McGladdery SL, 375
McGregor M, 457
McIlroy WE, 806
McIntyre NJ, 696
McKenna RJ Sr, 294
McKenna TJ, 194
McLaughlin JR, 105
McLellan TL, 654
McMath JC, 66
McNally D, 797
McSweeney M, 463
Meagher T, 510
Medical Research Council, 649
Medvei VC, 701
Meehan JP, 468
Meeks GR, 563
Meidl EJ, 499
Meissner H-H, 100
Mellinkoff SM, 459
Mellow AM, 698
Melnick J, 481
Melton LJ III, 466

Mendez MF, 735
Meno F, 367
Meroz N, 861
Messerli FH, 132
Metheny N, 463
Metzler C, 287
Meyer CT, 462
Meyer T, 375
Meyer TE, 455, 457
Meyerowitz BR, 460
Meyers DG, 385
Meyers MA, 479
Michi K-i, 279
Michie C, 500
Miles JE, 77
Milhorn HT Jr, 81
Miller A, 411
Miller AB, 298
Miller CS, 252
Miller MH, 187
Milzman DP, 117
Minasian H, 306
Minato S, 794
Minkin W, 205
Mitchell TL, 85
Mizuno A, 281
Model D, 211
Mollan RAB, 591
Molloy DW, 693, 806
Money BE, 240
Moodley J, 565
Mooij JJ, 212
Moore MJ, 258
Morley JE, 106
Morris JG, 682
Morrow F, 267
Morton ME, 283
Moses VK, 356
Moss AJ, 133
Moss R, 733
Moss SE, 238
Mozes M, 450
Mozes MF, 450
Muchmore EA, 101
Muehrcke RC, 207
Mueller EJ, 542
Mufti R al, 448
Mulley GP, 108

Mulrow CD, 313, 346
Munetz MR, 668
Muragh J, 278
Murphy RL Jr, 311, 326, 327
Murray HW, 831
Murray PI, 228
Murtagh J, 598, 606, 630
Musset de, 401
Muzaffar S, 89
Myllyla VV, 653

N

Najmaldin A, 554
Nakajima ST, 568
Napodano RJ, 866
Nardone DA, 10, 11, 64, 871
Nassar ME, 349
Nath AR, 330, 331
Nathanson M, 17
Nayak USL, 714
Naylor CD, 31, 501
Nelson KR, 669, 686
Nelson RS, 319
Nepp M, 573
Netland PA, 219
Neumann MJ, 462
Nevitt MC, 719
Newman L, 564
Newton JA, 190
Newton RW, 678
Niaz U, 690
Nieman LZ, 867
Niewoehner CB, 308
Ninia JG, 617
Nisar M, 334
Nishimura RA, 372
Noble H, 435
Noda S, 794
Nolting WE, 565
Nonino F, 113
Nordberg J, 202
Norman DC, 114
Norris JW, 428

Norton A, 759
Novack DH, 65
Nuriel H, 352
Nussenbatt RB, 766
Nuttall FQ, 308
Nzeako UC, 779

O

Oboler SK, 32
O'Brien MD, 747
Occupational and Environmental Health Committee of the American Lung Association of San Diego and Imperial Counties, 72
O'Connell EJ, 344
Odajnyk CM, 777
Oddone EZ, 868
Odom NJ, 473
O'Donnell AE, 819
Ogilvie CM, 329
Ogren JM, 121
O'Keeffe ST, 624, 746
Oldstone MB, 461
Oliphant M, 479
Olive KE, 395
Olofinboba KA, 602
O'Mara K, 438, 440
O'Neill TW, 362
Ono K, 670
O'Reilly S, 492
Orinius E, 387
O'Rourke KS, 608
O'Rourke RA, 355, 369, 394, 415
Orth G, 547
Orton D, 27
Osher RH, 236
Ostbye T, 430, 433
Ostick G, 707
O'Sullivan J, 451
Oung CO, 476
Owen WF Jr, 821

P

Paauw DS, 756
Palac DM, 10
Palestine AG, 764
Palmer RM, 140
Palmer RN, 580
Papadakis M, 481
Parish LC, 163
Park S, 178
Parrino TA, 363
Patel SR, 337, 339
Paton A, 78
Payne JE, 465
Paz LR de la, 396
Pearson CM, 634
Pearson MG, 329, 334
Peckham MJ, 86
Peeling WB, 537
Peipert JF, 566
Peitzman SJ, 131
Peller PA, 421
Pelletier G, 788
Peltier LF, 607
Penney DG, 20, 22
Perkin GD, 46
Perkins F, 120
Perloff D, 134
Perloff JK, 350, 412
Perry GY, 373
Peter JB, 634
Peters L, 810
Peterson DS, 792
Peterson MC, 12
Petty TL, 42
Pfleiderer AG, 247
Phanthumchinda K, 688
Phanuphak P, 688
Phelan JA, 772
Phillips CI, 241
Phillips JH, 389
Phillips SF, 466
Phillips TJ, 162
Pierson JC, 798
Piette WW, 185
Piha J, 141
Piirila P, 332, 333

Pilgrim C, 295
Pincus SH, 576
Pines A, 715
Pirie AM, 842
Pitegoff G, 718
Pitlik S, 373
Platt FW, 66
Polano MK, 161
Polley HF, 592
Poole A, 390
Poole-Wilson PA, 410
Porta J, 35
Pozderac RV, 614
Prema K, 272
Preston DS, 165
Prewitt LM, 158
Price RC, 722
Priebe WM, 464
Primrose RB, 567
Protheroe D, 583
Prout WG, 447
Pryor JP, 748
Psaty BM, 727
Puolijoki H, 155
Putsch RW III, 71
Puxty JA, 749
Pye M, 724
Pynsent PB, 597

Q

Quarry-Piggott VM, 381
Quesenberry CP Jr, 535, 539
Quigley C, 612
Quill TE, 866
Quincke, 401
Quinn M, 842
Qureshi B, 825

R

Rabhan NB, 205
Rachootin P, 660
Radack K, 178
Radwany SM, 154

Raife M, 556
Raiha I, 141
Rainey JB, 518
Raizada V, 402
Ramirez B, 274
Ramoska EA, 573
Rao PS, 288
Rapp CE Jr, 784
Ratzan RM, 549
Rault R, 852
Ray V, 541
Ray WF, 675
Rayos G, 413
Reddy PS, 367
Redman JF, 548
Reed CA, 429
Rees TS, 727
Reeves AG, 658
Reevss RA, 135
Regan WM, 702
Reilly DT, 605
Reinfeld H, 671
Reinke DB, 444
Reisman G, 801
Requena C, 197
Requena L, 197
Resnick NM, 586
Reuler JB, 871
Rhodes AR, 172
Ribeiro JP, 156
Rich EC, 240
Rich MW, 154
Rickman LS, 319, 513, 514
Riegelman RK, 43
Ries AL, 158
Rigel DS, 169, 170
Riley TL, 675
Ringenberg QS, 186
Rizzo C, 709
Robers LR, 214
Roberts KJ, 320
Roberts R, 693
Robins LN, 708
Robinson JK, 872
Rocco MB, 156
Roche J, 811
Rockwell S, 74

Rodriguez FR, 542
Roederer GO, 725
Rohde P, 855
Roman MJ, 128
Rosemberg SK, 550, 555
Rosen L, 527
Rosenberg SA, 835
Rosenfeld JB, 373
Rosenthal RN, 79
Roth JL, 264, 458
Rothenberg MH, 611
Rothman A, 374
Rourke JT, 544
Rousseau P, 716
Roy CR II, 556
Roy RR, 805
Rubenstein LZ, 140
Rubin J, 201
Rudzinski M, 790
Ruffin R, 660

S

Sabin S, 98
Sabra A, 635
Sacchetti AD, 573
Sackett DL, 13, 14, 434, 508
Sagebiel RW, 171
Sahn SA, 316
St. Clair EW, 868
Salopek TG, 164
Saltzman BR, 772
Salvatore R, 127
Samit AM, 260
Samsa GP, 214
Samuel D, 179
Sanchez M, 197
Sanders RM, 568
Sanders VR, 151
Sanes JN, 676
Santamaria J, 673
Sapira JD, 26, 47, 144, 242, 321, 398, 401, 502, 812, 813
Sarbah S, 775
Sareli P, 455

Suurmond D, 161
Svetkey LP, 493
Swan HJC, 416
Swartz WH, 575
Szasz G, 77
Szilagyi A, 476

T

Taft TN, 636
Tager RM, 832
Tajik AJ, 372
Takahashi K, 279
Tala E, 155
Talbot T, 275
Talbot W, 225
Talley NJ, 466
Tamayo SG, 513
Tambeur LJMT, 470
Tan L-B, 375
Tanaka DJ, 335
Tandberg D, 122
Tardiff K, 874
Teece MA, 532
Tei C, 730
ten Kate RW, 770
Teng EL, 781
Tennant F, 817
Ternouth I, 775
Thomas RJ, 659
Thompson BT, 343
Thompson HS, 231
Thompson IM, 542
Thomson WH, 475, 490
Thorpe KE, 434
Tierney LM Jr, 95
Timmis AJ, 383
Tinetti ME, 741
Tiver KW, 303
Tobin JN, 409
Tobin MJ, 153
Tombaugh TN, 696
Tomera KM, 553
Toole JF, 429
Tornelli JL, 85
Traboulsi EI, 244
Trebich C, 593

Truelove EL, 837
Tsapatsaris NP, 624
Tsementzis SA, 655
Tuazon CU, 831
Turnbull JM, 494
Turner G, 710
Turner MLC, 577
Tutschka PJ, 836
Tyberg TI, 424
Tyden G, 579

U

Uhlmann RF, 727
Ulbrecht JS, 619
Underwood KL, 735
United States Public
    Health Service, 33
Urbani CE, 296

V

Valacio R, 746
Valenti AJ, 769
Valori RM, 97
van Bijsterveld OP, 851
Van Bruggen AC, 212
Van den Hoogen HMM,
    600
van der Waal I, 770
Van Dooren BT, 212
Van Eijk JTM, 600
van Gool WA, 808
Van Hoven J, 679
Van Peenen HJ, 16
Van Ruiswyk, 435
Vaquer RA, 776
Varhaug JE, 286
Vaughan SC, 859
Venencie PY, 179
Venner RM, 601
Ventura HO, 132
Verghese A, 93, 104, 208,
    506, 662
Viganotti G, 297

Vine DL, 384
Visintin J-M, 127

W

Waal I van der, 770
Waddell G, 601
Wagner G, 560
Wakefield DS, 150
Waks AU, 840
Walker A, 744
Walker HK, 48, 203
Walker JEC, 276
Walker JM, 444
Wallace C, 285
Wallace GB, 678
Wallis LA, 572, 874
Walsh DB, 658
Walshaw MJ, 334
Walshe TM, 750
Walstra GJM, 808
Walzak MP, 549
Walzer A, 495
Wang K, 376
Wang Q, 238
Ward C, 142
Wasserman SS, 119
Wassertheil-Smoller S,
    409
Watanakunakorn C, 123
Watkinson JC, 30
Watson YI, 697
Waugh RA, 868
Wee AS, 674
Wehrle MA, 463
Wei JY, 397
Weinert M, 771
Weinstein C, 187
Weiss NS, 136, 535
Wellens HJ, 353
Weller MP, 700
Welsh J, 706
Wenrich MD, 756
Werner SC, 226
Wertheimer AJ, 845
Wescott WB, 263
Weston CF, 391

Weston WW, 54-56
Westreich LM, 79
Wheeler L, 560
Wheeler RA, 557
Wheeler SD, 853
Whitehouse PJ, 691
Whitfield H, 585
Wiener S, 17
Wiener SL, 310, 356, 357, 359
Wiernik PH, 838
Wiersma L, 463
Wild K, 500
Wilken MK, 385
Williams DR, 82
Williams JW Jr, 213, 214, 483
Williams R, 505, 512
Williamson DL, 502
Willms JL, 49
Wilson JD, 309
Wilson JR, 413
Wilson T, 556
Wilt TJ, 530
Winawer SJ, 536
Winchester DP, 294

Wing S, 380
Winograd CH, 719
Wise MP, 684
Witkowski JA, 163
Witte CL, 603
Witte MH, 603
Wolfe JHN, 605
Wolff K, 160
Wolfkiel CJ, 357
Wolf-Klein GP, 699
Wolgamuth BR, 265
Wong M, 730
Wood NK, 253
Woodruff GHA, 793
Woods B O'B, 624
Wooley AC, 109
Woska D, 404
Wray NP, 19
Wynne JM, 847

Y

Yaffe ME, 785
Yajima T, 157
Yamaguchi K, 281

Yamase H, 268
Yang JC, 514
Yee J, 632
Yeh M, 114
Yeoh TK, 413
Yurchak PM, 860

Z

Zamora-Quezada JC, 818
Zatouroff M, 626
Zavala DC, 361
Zema MJ, 420
Ziegler DK, 650
Zitelli BJ, 50
Zive MA, 245
Zoli M, 507
Zorc TG, 819
Zornow DH, 558
Zweifler AJ, 137

Subject Index

Note: Numbers following entries are for references, not pages.

A

Abdomen, 458-464
  acute, 468-475
    Cullen's and Grey Turner's signs in, 476-479
    left lower vs. right upper quadrant pain, 561
    medical history and therapeutic choices, 87
    rectal examination and, 518, 519
  ascites, 480-483
  chronic symptoms, 484-490
  kidneys and renal vasculature, 491-495
  liver and gallbladder, 496-507
  patient history, 465-467
  radiography, digital rectal examination and, 753
  spleen, 508-514
  urinary bladder, 515-517
Abdominal aortic aneuyrsm, 441-444, 549
Abdominal pressure test, 370, 441
Abdominal wall tenderness, 488-490
Abdominojugular test, 408, 452, 453
Acanthosis nigricans, 177
Achilles tendon reflex, 679, 683
Achondroplasia, brain stem compression in, 153
Acid reflux, dental erosion and, 274
Acne, polycystic ovaries and, 190
Acquired immune deficiency syndrome; *see* Human immunodeficiency virus infection and AIDS

Acrochordons, multiple, 177
Activities of daily living, assessing, 63
Addiction, 812, 813; *see also* Alcohol abuse; Drug abuse
Addison's disease, 593
Adie's syndrome, 215
Adolescents, 784; *see also* Pediatrics
  alcoholism in, 786, 788-790
  anorexia and bulimia in, 791, 792
  rectal examination in, 785
Advance directives, 83
Age of patient, stated, 103
Aging; *see also* Geriatrics
  cardiac sounds and, 367
  third heart sound and, 385
AIDS; *see* Human immunodeficiency virus infection and AIDS
Akathisia, drug-induced, 664
Albumin, fingernails and, 207
Alcohol abuse
  in adolescents, 786, 788-790
  in elderly, 706, 710
  fetal alcohol syndrome, 787
  in patient history, 78
Alcohol pain, in Hodgkin's disease, 86
Allen test, 438, 440
Alpha-transforming growth factor, 177
Alveolitis, fibrosing, crackles in, 328, 332, 334
Alzheimer's disease, 802, 803, 806
  clock drawing in, 698, 699, 735
Amaurosis fugax, 234
American Sign Language, 800

Baker's cyst, ruptured, 612, 614
Balance, in elderly, 714
Ballet dancers, 679
Basal body temperature, 841
Basal cell carcinoma of anus, 528
Battered woman syndrome, 844
Bicycle test of van Gelderen, 595
Bilingual consultation, 822, 823
Bismuth intoxication, 700
Black patients with AIDS, 763
Bladder, 515-517
Bleeding
  nail bed, 798
  retinal, 236
  subungual splinter, 180
Blindness, 724
Blinking and release reflexes, 659
Blood depletion, 107; see also Volume status assessment
Blood pressure, 124-137
  heart rate and pulse character, 145-149
  measurement, 124-126, 134, 135, 138, 840
  orthostatic pulse and hypotension and, 138-142
  pulsus paradoxus, 143, 144
Blood pressure cuffs, 369, 840
Blue scrotum sign of Bryant, 549
Blue toe syndrome, 624
Body temperature, 113-123
  basal, 841
Bone marrow transplantation, 834, 836, 837
Bowel disease, 465-467
Bowel sounds, 469, 799
Brachioradial delay, 436
Brain computed tomography, in alcohol withdrawal seizures, 789
Brain stem compression, in achondroplasia, 153
Breast cancer
  axillary node palpation in, 286
  localized mastalgia as presenting symptom in, 297
  and mimics and fibrocystic conditions, 298-306
Breast implants, physical examination and, 293

Breasts
  aberrant mammary tissue and nephrourinary malignancy, 296
  cultural resistance to exposure, 826
  examination, 290-295, 305
    in cancer screening, 298, 729
    in obese patients, 839
  gynecomastia, 307-309
Breathing; see also Respiratory system
  apneustic, 153
  periodic, 155-157
Bronchial stenosis, 318
Bronchiectasis, crackles in, 332
Brudzinski's sign, 662, 749
Bruits
  abdominal, 491, 494
  carotid, 428-430, 434
    differentiation from other disorders, 277
  in elderly, 435
  hemodialysis and, 852, 853
  hepatic rub and, 504
Bryant's blue scrotum sign, 549
Buerger's test, 447
Bulimia, 791
Bursitis, 587
Butterfly sign, 179

C

CAGE questionnaire, 706
Calcium, 191, 853
Calluses, cocaine abuse and, 814
Calves, deep venous thrombosis, 612
Canadian National Breast Screening Study, 298
Cancer; see also specific organs
  detection by physical examination, 33
  genetics and, 80
  supraclavicular metastasis, 289
Cancer therapy patients, 834
Candidal infection, oral, 836
Capillary refill, 102, 112
Cardiac auscultation, 364-368
  maneuvers and manipulations, 369-376
  murmurs, 386-397
  second heart sound, 377

Cardiac auscultation–*cont'd*
  teaching, 867
  third and fourth heart sounds, 378-385
Cardiac disorders; *see* Heart, specific settings and conditions
Cardiac tamponade, pulsus paradoxus in, 143
Cardiac transplantation, 156
Cardiomegaly, 356, 362
Cardiopulmonary arrest, 150
Cardiovascular disease, periodic breathing in, 157
Cardiovascular system; *see also* Heart; Peripheral vasculature
  palpation, 363
Carotid arteries, 428-435
Carotid artery stenosis, 234
Carotid bruits, 428-430, 434
  differentiation from other disorders, 277
  in elderly, 435
Carotid endartertectomy, 243
Carpal tunnel syndrome, 628, 635
Cartilage, knee, 608
Carvallo sign, 370
Case presentation, 856-860
Catheterization, right-heart, 417
Cat-scratch disease, in AIDS, 762
Cauda equina compression, 595
Central venous pressure, abnormal, 452
Cerebral function, 656-659; *see also* Mental status and psychiatric evaluation
Cervical auscultation, 22
Cervical cord damage, 670
Cervical disc rupture, 665
Cervical myelopathy, 682
Cervical nodes, lymph, palpable, 287
Cervix
  abnormalities and cancer, screening for, 565, 566, 751
  and uterus examination, 559-572
Chaperones, 580-583
Cheilitis, 270, 275
Chemical warfare, skin lesions from, 197
Chemotherapy, oral manifestations, 834

Chest examination; *see also* Respiratory system
  foam sponge as teaching aid in, 861
  physical signs in, 315
Cheyne-Stokes respiration, 155-157
Chief complaint, 60
Child abuse, sexual, 846, 847
Children; *see* Pediatrics
Choroiditis in AIDS, 765
Chronic fatigue syndrome, 266
Chronic obstructive pulmonary disease, 332, 335, 338; *see also* Obstructive airways disease
Cirrhosis, 179, 308
Clavicular auscultation, 396
Clinical examination; *see* Examination
Clock drawing, 697-699, 734, 735
Closed eyes sign, 471, 472
Clubbing
  hypertrophic osteoarthopathy and, 202, 776
  Schamroth's sign in, 206
  from secondary hyperparathyroidism, 201
Cobalamin deficiency, 681
Cocaine abuse, 814-816, 818
Coffee cup sign, 633
Cognition in HIV patients, 781
Cognitive capacity, 694; *see also* Mental status and psychiatric evaluation
Colonoscopy, 465
Colon polyps, skin tags and, 178
Colorectal cancer, fecal occult blood testing, 531-536
Comatose and unresponsive patients, 793, 794
Communication
  case presentation, 856-860
  in critical illness, 795
  culture and, 71, 822-827
  interviewing and history-taking, 51-83
  verbal instructions on blood pressure measurement, 125
Competence, in interviewing, 66
Computed tomography, in alcohol withdrawal seizures, 789
Concentration, loss of, 692

Concentration camp survivors, 848
Congestive heart failure, 403-405, 408, 409, 412, 413
  ocular finds, 220
  symptoms, 40
  third heart sound in, 380
Conjunctivitis, 224, 225, 227
Connective tissue diseases, nailfold capillary microscopy in, 204
Constrictive pericarditis, pericardial knock in, 424
Consultations, 9
COPD; see Chronic obstructive pulmonary disease; Obstructive airways disease
Corneal arcus, 725
Coronary artery surgery, blood pressure measurement before, 124
Coughing test, in peritonitis, 470
Courvoisier's law, 506
Crack cocaine, free-basing, 818
Crackles, 323, 328-334, 405, 406
Cranial nerves, 660
Crescent sign, 614
Creutzfeldt-Jakob disease, 803
Crimson crescents, 266
Critical care unit patients, 795-799
Crohn's disease, 275
Cullen's sign and variants, 476-479
Cultural differences, 69, 71, 822-827
Cyanosis, 99
Cystic fibrosis, 551
Cysts
  Baker's, ruptured, 612, 614
  polycystic kidney disease, 296
  polycystic ovaries, 190
  popliteal cyst rupture, 612
Cytomegalovirus retinitis, 764, 767

D

Date rape, 844
Dco, crackles and, 405
Deep venous thrombosis, 612
Dehydration, in elderly, 108, 109
Delirium, 690
Dementia
  clock drawing in, 697-699

Dementia–cont'd
  in elderly, 731-735
  evaluation, 690-692, 802-804, 806-808
Dental erosion
  in acid reflux disease, 274
  in bulimia, 791
  in cocaine users, 815, 816
Dentures, 728
Depression, in AIDS, 755
De Quervain's tenosynovitis, 630
Dermatology; see Skin
Dermatomyositis, 204
Dermatoses, vulvar, 576
Diabetes mellitus
  cutaneous manifestations, 191
  family history and risk of complications, 82
  foot disease in, 619, 620
  juvenile, fibrous disease of breast in, 299
Diabetic neuropathy, sensory examination in, 641
Diagnosis, 34-43; see also Examination; Interviewing and history-taking
  contributions of history, physical examination, and laboratory diagnosis to, 12
  cultural barriers in, 69
  housestaff skill assessment with cardiology patient simulator, 868
  morgues as classroom for, 873
  olfactory, 23
  taught in nursing home, 863, 870
Diastolic pressure, criteria for, 133
Diastolic sounds and murmurs, in mitral valve prolapse, 397
Differential collapsing pulses, 451
Difficult interviews, 68-71, 583, 862
Difficult patients, 809, 854, 855
Diffusing capacity of carbon monoxide, crackles and, 405
Digital clubbing, 201, 202, 206
Digital rectal examination; see Prostate examination, per rectum; Rectal examination
Digiti quinti sign, 663
Disability, 810
  simulated, 832

Disc rupture, 665
Doppler echocardiography
    in aortic insufficiency, 40
    in aortic regurgitation, 399
    in aortic stenosis, 386, 388
    in regurgitant lesions, 393
Draw-a-Clock test, 734; *see also* Clock
    drawing
Drawer sign in ankle, 613
Drinking disorders; *see* Alcohol abuse
Drug abuse, 79, 811-819
Dyskinesia, respiratory, 154
Dyspepsia, nonulcer, 466
Dysphagia, stethoscopes in, 22
Dysplastic nevi, 170-172
Dyspnea, 87
    congestive heart failure diagnosis in,
        408
    discriminating causes of, 346
    heart and lung involvement in, 420
    patient history, 310

E

Earlobe crease, 245, 246
Ear oximetry, 158
Ears, 245-250
Ear thermometry, 117, 118
Ecchmosis, 614, 718
Echocardiography
    in aortic insufficiency, 40
    in aortic regurgitation, 399
    in aortic stenosis, 386, 388
    in mitral valve prolapse, 395
    in regurgitant lesions, 393
Edema
    breast, 302
    hypoproteinemic, 615
    myoedema in paralytic rabies, 688
    pitting, 198
    pretibial myxedema, 616
    scrotal, 554
Edentulous elderly patient, 728
Education, bedside skills teaching, 861-
    874
Egophony, 321
Elbow, tennis, 633
Elderly; *see* Geriatrics

Elephantiasis nostras, 602
Emboli
    retinal cholesterol, 233, 243
    talc, of retinal vessels, 811
Embolism, pulmonary, high fever in, 123-
    124
Emergency department, pelvic examina-
    tion in, 561
Emesis, 88
    in anorexia and bulimia, 791, 792
Empathy, 51
Endocarditis, infectious, 631, 632
Endocrine diseases, skin signs and involve-
    ment in, 190-194
End-stage renal disease, 849-853
Enoxaparin-induced skin necrosis, 196
Enteral feeding tubes, 462, 463
Epigastric tenderness, 464
Epistaxis, hypertension and, 136
Erythrocyte sedimentation rate, 600
Erythromelalgia, 622
Erythroplasia, 261
Esophagus, aphthous ulcers of, 769
Ethnic differences, 69, 71, 822-827
Examination, 1-19; *see also specific organ
        systems and disorders*
    complete annual, 4
    errors, 17
    ethnicity and, 824-827
    in intensive care unit, 796, 797
    methods, 20-30
    nutritional assessment, 105, 106
    physical, general, 91-104
    precision and accuracy in, 13
    reference standards, 31
    screening, 32, 33
    technology and physical diagnosis, 34-
        43
    textbooks, 44-50
    volume status assessment, 107-112
Exercise, in heart failure, 156
Exophthalmos, in congestive heart failure,
    220
Extremities, 590, 676; *see also* Locomotor
        system and limbs; Lower limb;
        Upper limb
Eye disorders
    in HIV patients, 764-767
    pupils, 227-232

Eye disorders–*cont'd*
    retina, 233-244
Eye examination, 215, 217
    in elderly, 725
    external eye, 219-226
    textbooks, 216, 218

F

Face and head, 209-213
Facial ecchymoses, 718
Facial expression, in appendicitis, 473
Facial pain, patient history, 651
Falls, in elderly, 714, 718
Family history, 80-82
Fatigue (chronic fatigue syndrome), crimson crescents in, 266
Fecal occult blood testing, 531-536
Feet, 618-626
Femur fractures, 607
Fetal alcohol syndrome, 787
Fever; *see also* Temperature
    in acute stroke, 113
    factitious, 831
    in pulmonary embolism, 123-124
    rash and, 189
    of unknown origin, in elderly, 720
Fibromyalgia syndrome, 652
Fibrosing alveolitis, crackles in, 328, 332, 334
Fibrosis, pulmonary, 329
Fibrous disease of breast, in juvenile diabetes, 299
Finger clubbing, 201, 202, 206
Fingernails; *see* Nails
Finger pads, tophaceous deposition in, 637
Finkelstein's test, 629, 630
Flexion contractures, dementia and, 807
Fluid in knee, 610
Foam sponge, as teaching aid, 861
Folstein Mini-Mental State Examination;
    see Mini-Mental State Examination
Foot, 618-626
Foot pulse palpation, 445, 446, 448, 449
Forced expiratory time, 337-340
Fourth heart sound, 378, 381, 384

Fractures
    hip and femur, 607
    mandibular, 254
    nasal, 718
    osteoporotic compression, of thoracic vertebrae, 738
    skull, 209
Friction rubs, 421-423
Frostbite, in homeless persons, 820
Fundus examination, 241-242, 804

G

Gag reflex in disease, 660
Gait disorders
    in elderly, 739, 740
    hysterical, 828
Gait mechanisms, 675
Gallbladder, enlarged, 506
Gardner's syndrome, 244
Gastrocnemius compression sign, 450
Gastroesophageal reflux disease, dental erosion and, 274
Gastrointestinal disease, 178, 179
    oral manifestations, 264
Gay patients, 821
Genetics, cancer and, 80
Genital examination, female; *see also*
    Pelvic examination and gynecologic evaluation
    teaching associates and, 874
Genital examination, male, 544-558
Genograms, 81
Geographic tongue, 263
Geriatrics, 703-705
    aortic regurgitation, 399
    aortic stenosis, 386
    appearance and functional assessment, 712-713, 715-717, 719
    body temperature, 114
    breasts, 729
    carotid bruits, 435
    dehydration, 108, 109
    eye examination, 725
    falls, 714, 718
    fourth heart sound, 381

Heart failure–*cont'd*
  periodic breathing during exercise in,
    156
  third heart sound of, 380, 382
Heart murmurs, 386-397; *see* Murmurs
  in elderly, 730
  left-sided regurgitant, 369
  in renal failure, 849, 852
  of tricuspid regurgitation, 370
Heart rate, pulse character and, 145-149
Heel pain, 618
Hemarthrosis with synovial rupture, 614
Hematocolpos, 754
Hematologic disorders, skin signs and
    involvement in, 180-187
Hematomas
  from pen pressing, 798
  subdural, 644, 673
Hemiparesis, 663, 672
  hysterical, 830
Hemoccult test, 532, 533
Hemodialysis, bruits and, 852, 853
Hemodynamics, in congestive heart fail-
    ure, 412
Hemoglobin, reduced, 99
Hemorrhage
  nail bed, 798
  retinal, 236
  subungual splinter, 180
Henoch-Schönlein purpura, 185
Hepatic pressure maneuver, 370
Hepatitis B, 640, 686
Hepatojugular reflux test (abdominojugu-
    lar test), 370, 408, 452, 453
Hernia, laughing hernia sign, 544
Herpes simplex lesions, perianal ulcera-
    tive, 779, 780
High blood pressure; *see* Hypertension
Hip flexion-abduction, in asterixis, 794
Hips, 606, 607
Hirsutism, screening for sinister causes,
    194
History; *see* Interviewing and history taking
HIV; *see* Human immunodeficiency virus
    infection and AIDS
Hodgkin's disease, 86
Hollenhorst plaques, 233, 243
Holocaust survivors, 848
Homeless persons, 820

Homosexual patients, 821
Hooking maneuver, 361
Hostile patients, 809
Human immunodeficiency virus infection
    and AIDS, 755-758
  anorectal and genital area, 779, 780
  cognition, 781
  eyes, 764-767
  hypertrophic osteoarthropathy, 776
  limbs and locomotor system, 777, 778
  lymph nodes, 773-775
  mouth and face, 768-772
  pulmonary abnormalities, 319
  skin, nails, and hair, 188, 759-763
Human papillomavirus
  female infection, 565, 566
  male infection, 547, 550, 555
Hymen, imperforate, 568
Hyperalgesic pseudothrombophlebitis, 777
Hypercapnia, 100
Hyperparathyroidism, secondary, 201
Hypertension
  diagnosis, 135
  renovascular, 491, 493, 494
  retinopathy and, 238
  symptoms and, 136
  vascular disease in, auscultatory gap
    and, 128
Hypertrophic osteoarthropathy
  in AIDS, 776
  clubbing and, 202
  pulmonary, 198
Hyperventilation syndrome, 155
Hypoalbuminemia, fingernails in, 207
Hypoproteinemic edema, 615
Hypotension, 138-142
  postexertional, 129
  postprandial, 130, 131
  volume status and, 107-108, 110-112
Hypothyroidism, 684
Hypovolemia, 112; *see also* Volume status
    assessment
Hysteria, 828-830

I

Immigrants, 824, 827, 843
Immobility, in elderly, 712, 741

Immunodeficiency, oral hairy leukoplakia
  and, 268
Imperforate hymen, 568
Implants, breast, physical examination and,
  293
Impotence, sexual history in, 76
Incontinence, urinary, 584-586
Infectious disease
  bacterial meningitis, 661
  endocarditis, 631, 632
  HIV; see Human immunodeficiency
    virus infection and AIDS
  lateral slump sign in, 716
  papillomavirus
    female infection, 565, 566
    male infection, 547, 550, 555
  presentation in granulocytopenic
    patients, 838
  screening in internationally adopted
    child, 824
  skin involvement in, 188, 189
Infrared emission detection thermometry,
  in acute otitis media, 117
Infrared tympanic thermometer, 117, 118,
  120
Intensive care unit, examination in, 796, 797
Interleukin-2, 835
Intermittent positive pressure ventilation,
  799
Interstitial lung disease, crackles in, 328
Interviewing and history-taking, 8, 51-67;
  see also specific disorders
  accuracy of history, 62
  competence in, 66
  core curriculum for residencies in inter-
    nal medicine, 866
  difficult interviews, 68-71, 583, 862
  in elderly, 706-711
  family history, 80-82
  functions of history, 65
  in making medical diagnosis, 12
  occupational history, 72
  patient interrogation and rhinoscopy,
    251
  in pregnancy, 573
  sexual history, 73-77
  substance abuse, 78, 79

Interviewing and history-taking–cont'd
  symptoms and syndromes, 86-90
  systems review, 84, 85
  values history, 83
Intracranial tumor noises, 212
Intraocular pressure, 219, 220
Intravenous drug abuse, 811, 812, 819
Involuntary movements; see Movements,
  involuntary
Iritis, 227
Iron, oral, Hemoccult test and, 532, 533
Irritable bowel syndrome, 466, 484-487
Ischemia, lower limb, 447
Ischemic heart disease, 138, 414-418
Ischemic stroke, skin temperature in, 653
Ischemic ulcers, 446

J

Janeway lesion, 631
Jaundice, 506
Jogger's toe, 625
Joints, 591, 592; see also specific joints
Jugular venous distension, 403

K

Kaposi sarcoma, 188, 756, 762
Kernig's sign, 662, 749
Kidneys and renal vasculature, 491-495
Knees, 608-611
Korotkoff sounds IV and V, 842
Kussmaul's sign, 455-457
Kyphosis, 738

L

Language
  bilingual consultation, 822, 823
  in patient care, 53
Laparoscopy, fiberoptic, pelvic examina-
    tion vs., 571
Lateral nystagmus, 786
Lateral slump sign, 716, 717

Palpation–*cont'd*
    precordial, 355-358
    radial artery, 437
    scrotum, 558
    skin, 163
    spleen, 509, 512
    superficial temporal artery, 427
    thyroid gland, 284
    in tumor assessment, 30
    uterine artery pulsation, 563
    vas deferens, 551
Pancreatic graft failure, 579
Pancreatitis, signs in, 476, 478, 479
Papanicolaou smears, 565, 566, 751
Papillomaviral infection
    female, 565, 566
    male, 547, 550, 555
Paralytic rabies, myoedema in, 688
Paresthesias, in fibromyalgia syndrome, 652
Patellar surface irregularities, 609
Patient-centered interviewing, 54-56
Patients, hostile, 809
Pectoral crease, oblique, 669
Pedal pulse palpation, 445, 446, 448, 449
Pediatrics, 782-785
    alcoholism, 786-790
    physical diagnosis, 50
    screening for infectious disease, 824
    sexual abuse, 846, 847
Pelvic examination and gynecologic evaluation
    adnexal examination and findings, 578, 579
    in autism, 833
    chaperones in, 580-583
    in elderly, 751-752
    external (vulvar) examination, 576, 577
    patient history, 573
    positioning, 574, 575
    sexual history, 73
    teaching, 865
    transvaginal sonography vs., 36
    urinary incontinence, 584-586
    uterine and cervical examination, 559-572
Pelvic pain, cured by pelvic examination, 569, 570
Pemberton sign, 285
Penis, 545-550

Pentamidine, 778
Pen torch (penlight) test, 227, 228
Peptic ulcer disease, 464, 707
Percussion, 21-26, 320; *see also* Auscultatory percussion
    of left cardiac border, 360
    precordial, 356-359
    spleen, 509, 510, 512
Perianal herpes lesions, 779, 780
Pericardial disease, 421-424, 455
Perimylolysis, 791
Periodic breathing, 155-157
Peripheral nerve injuries, 649
Peripheral vasculature
    arteries, 425-451
    veins, 452-457
Peritonitis, coughing test in, 470
Pernicious anemia, 183
Personality, type A, 418
Pharynx, aphthous ulcers of, 769
Phalen sign, 628
Pheochromocytoma, mental symptoms in, 701
pH of aspirated fluid, in enteral feeding tube placement, 462
Physical examination, 91-104; *see also* Examination
Physical findings, 5, 11
Physically challenged persons, 810
Pigmented and melanocytic lesions, 166-173
Pis-en-deux, 585
Pitting edema, 198
Pituitary disease, cutaneous manifestations, 191
Plantar fasciitis, 618
Plantar reflexes, 679, 744
Pleural effusion, 317
Plunging ranula, 281
Pneumocystis carinii, in AIDS, 776, 778
Pneumomediastinum, 316
Pneumonia, crackles in, 333
Pneumophonography, 333
Pneumothorax, 316
Podalgia, 618, 621
Polycystic kidney disease, 296
Polycystic ovaries, acne and, 190
Polyps, colon, skin tags and, 178
Popliteal cyst rupture, 612

Porphyria, dermatologic manifestations, 182
Positioning, in pelvic examination, 574, 575
Postexertional hypotension, 129
Postmenopausal palpable ovary syndrome, 578
Postprandial hypotension, 130, 131
Postural hypotension; *see* Orthostatic hypotension
Posture
    crackles and, 406
    lying obliquely across bed, 715, 717
    in spinal stenosis, 599
Precordial motion, 354
Precordial palpation and percussion, 355-358, 360
Pregnancy
    hypertensive, 842
    ovulation detection, 841
    palpable uterine artery pulsation in, 563
    patient history in, 573
    ruptured extrauterine, 477
Premature ventricular complex, 376
Pretibial myxedema, 616
Progressive systemic sclerosis, 204
Pronus angina, 352
Proportional pulse pressure, 413
Prostate cancer, 539-543
Prostate examination, per rectum, 537-543
Prostate-specific antigen, 538
Prosthetic valves, normally functioning, auscultation of, 402
Protein C deficiency, 181
Pruritus vulvae, 576
PSA, 538
Pseudocoma, 793
Pseudogoiter, 283
Pseudohypertension, 137
    Osler's maneuver and, 127, 132
Pseudoseizures, 687, 793
Pseudothrombophlebitis, hyperalgesic, 777
Pseudothrombophlebitis syndrome, 612
Psoriasis, 195
Psychiatric evaluation and mental status, 690-702
    in elderly, 715, 717, 731-735
    in HIV patients, 781
Psychiatric interviews, chaperones in, 583

Psychoneurosis, 97
Psychosocial factors, in interview, 70
Pulmonary diffusing capacity, in left ventricle dysfunction, 406
Pulmonary embolism, high fever in, 123-124
Pulmonary examination, 311-346; *see also* Lung sounds; Respiratory system
Pulmonary osteoarthropathy, hypertrophic, 198
Pulmonary patients, office evaluation, 94
Pulse
    character, 145-149
    differential collapsing pulses, 451
    orthostatic, 138-142
    pedal, palpation, 445, 446, 448, 449
Pulse oximetry, 158, 438-440
Pulsus alternans, 145
Pulsus paradoxus, 143, 144
Pupils, 227-232, 241
Purpura fulminans, 181
Pyopneumothorax, bilateral, 819

R

Rabies, paralytic, myoedema in, 688
Race, 822-827
Radial artery palpation, 437
Radiculopathy, lumbar entrapment, 667
Radiography, abdominal, digital rectal examination and, 753
Rales, 405; *see also* Crackles
Rape, 844, 845
Rapid eye test, in drug abuse detection, 817
Rash, 187, 189
Raynaud's disease, 204
Rectal cancer, 525, 528
    fecal occult blood testing, 531-536
Rectal examination, 518-530
    in adolescent males, 785
    in elderly, 753-754
    in irritable bowel syndrome, 487
    prostate examination per rectum, 537-543
    teaching associates and, 874
Red eye, 225

Red eye–*cont'd*
    penlight test for, 227, 228
    in renal failure, 851
Reference standards, 31
Reflexes
    Achilles tendon, 679, 682
    in Alzheimer's disease, 806
    ankle jerks, 683, 745-748
    gag, in disease, 660
    patellar, 679
    release, 659
    scapulohumeral, 683
    slow relaxing, 684
Reflex sympathetic dystrophy, 654
Reflux disease, dental erosion and, 274
Regurgitant lesions, false-negative auscultation of, 393
Regurgitation
    aortic, 399, 401
    tricuspid, 370, 371
Release reflexes, 659
Renal cell carcinoma, 296, 556
Renal disease, end-stage, 849-853
Renal vasculature, 491-495
Respiration, Cheyne-Stokes, 155-157
Respiratory rate, in elderly, 722
Respiratory rate and pattern, 150-154
Respiratory system
    patient history, 310
    physical examination, 313-315
        basic science, 311, 312
        domains other than conventional
            lung sounds, 316-321
        lung sounds, 322-334
        obstructive airways disease, 335-346
Respiratory tract symptoms, in giant cell
    arteritis, 723
Retardation, 805
Retina, 233-244
Retinal vein, spontaneous pulsations of, 239
Retinal vessels, talc emboli of, 811
Retinitis in AIDS, 764, 765, 767
Rheumatic disease, foot examination in, 623
Rheumatologic examination, 589, 592
Rhinitis, allergic, 251
Rhinoscopy, patient interrogation and, 251
Right-heart catheterization, 417

Right iliac fossa squelch sign, 484
Right ventricle, infarction, 415

S

Sacroiliac tests, 594
Sarcoidosis, crackles in, 328
Scalp infarction, 724
Scalp soft tissue injury, 209
Scapular hump, 669
Scapulohumeral reflex, 683
Schamroth's sign, 206
Scleroderma, neck sign in, 280
Sclerosis, progressive systemic, 204
Scratch test, in liver examination, 497
Screening, 32, 33
    Alzheimer's disease, 699
    breast cancer, 298, 304, 729; *see also*
        Breasts, examination
    cervical abnormalities and cancer, 565, 566, 751
    cognitive capacity, 694
    colorectal cancer, 525, 531-536
    drinking disorders in elderly, 706
    functional disability in elderly, 713
    hearing in elderly, 726, 727
    heart examination, 348
    orthopedic, 588
    renovascular disease, 493
Scrotum
    blue scrotum sign of Bryant, 549
    edema, 554
    palpation, 558
Second heart sound, 377
Seizures
    in alcohol withdrawal, 789
    pseudoseizures, 687
    tongue biting in, 265
Sensory examination, 685, 686
    in diabetic peripheral neuropathy, 641
    small corks test, 687
    two-point discrimination test, 782
Serratoglossia, 276
Sexual abuse of children, 846, 847
Sexually transmitted diseases, 547, 548, 550, 555
Sheet sign in AIDS, 755
Shimizu reflex, 683

Shoulder disorders, 636
Shoulder displacement, in trapezius weakness, 669
Shoulder-pad sign, 634
Signs, 6; *see also* Vital signs
Sinus examination, 213, 214
Skin, 159-163
  color, ear oximetry and, 158
  enoxaparin-induced necrosis, 196
  facial, in smokers, 211
  in HIV patients, 188, 758, 760, 762
  infarction, cocaine abuse and, 818
  interleukin-2 and, 835
  mustard gas-induced lesions, 197
  pigmented and melanocytic lesions, 166-173
  psoriasis, 195
  in systemic disease
    endocrine diseases, 190-194
    gastrointestinal and hepatobiliary disorders, 178, 179
    general signs and neoplasia, 174-177
    vasculitides and hematologic disorders, 180-187
  temperature, in ischemic stroke, 653
  textbooks, 160, 161
  uremia complications, 852
  vulvar dermatoses and pruritus vulvae, 576
Skin cancer
  detection in clinical practice examination, 872
  malignant melanoma, 166, 167, 169, 170, 172, 173
  nonmelanocytic, 164, 165
Skull fracture, 209
Slipping rib syndrome, 361
Small corks test, 685
Smells, in diagnosis, 23
Smoker's face, 211
Smoking cessation, harlequin nail and, 208
Snout suffocation syndrome, 210
Spatula test, for mandibular fracture, 254
Sphygmomanometry, 126, 134, 144
Spine, 590, 594-600
  cervical cord damage, 670
  lumbar entrapment radiculopathy, 667

Splenomegaly, 508-514
Splinter hemorrhage, subungual, 180
Spondylitis, ankylosing, 35, 594, 600
Sponge, foam, as teaching aid, 861
Spoon test, 655
Sports injuries, 588, 633
Springing test for cervical rib identification, 288
Staff performance and error, 18, 19
Stare, in congestive heart failure, 220
Sternomastoid, in neck examination, 282
Stethoscopes, 2; *see also* Auscultation; Auscultatory percussion
  in abdominal examination, 460, 461
  acoustics, 20, 22
  defective, 27, 28
  in joint examination, 27, 28
Stethoscope sign, 459
Stiffness, 677
Stokes-Adams attack, vasovagal syncope vs., 230
Stomatitis, 101
Stoop-test, 667
Strangury, 585
Strength assessment, lower limb, 666
Stress test, four-step, in hip osteoarthritis, 606
Stroke
  clinical assessment, 643
  fever in, 113
  ischemic, skin temperature in, 653
Subclavian artery stenosis, 124
Subdural hematomas, 644, 673
Substance abuse; *see also* Alcohol abuse; Drug abuse
  in patient history, 78, 79
Sudomotor dysfunction, 655
Superficial temporal arteries, 427
Supraclavicular metastasis, 289
Swallowing sounds, detecting, 22, 279
Swollen leg, 605
Symptoms and syndromes, 86-90
Syndromes and symptoms, 86-90
Systemic lupus erythematosus, cutaneous manifestations, 187
Systems review, in patient history, 84, 85
Systolic murmurs, 390, 394

T

Tachypnea, in body temperature measurement, 122
Talc emboli of retinal vessels, 811
Tardive dyskinesia, 154
Teaching bedside skills, 861-874
Technology and physical diagnosis, 34-43
Teeth erosion
  in acid reflux disease, 274
  in bulimia, 791
  in cocaine users, 815, 816
Telangiectasias of anterior chest, 760
Telangiectatic veins, 617
Telephone interviewing and counseling, 59
Temperature
  body, 113-123
    basal, 841
    oral, in elderly, 721
  skin, in ischemic stroke, 653
  urinary, 831
Tendinitis, 587
Tennis elbow, 633
Tenosynovitis, De Quervain's, 630
Terry's nails, 203
Testes, 553, 556, 557
Textbooks
  neurologic examination, 642, 645, 646, 649
  ophthalmology, 216, 217
  oral disease, 252, 253
  otology, 248, 249
  physical examination, 44-50
  skin, 160, 161, 174, 176
α-TGF, 177
Thermometry, 117, 118, 120-122
Thigh pain or tenderness, 90
Third heart sound, 379, 380, 382-385
Thoracic vertebrae, osteoporotic compression fractures of, 738
Thrombosis, deep venous, 612
Thyroid disease
  autoimmune, 616
  cutaneous manifestations, 191
  Graves' ophthalmopathy and, 221
  hypothyroidism, 684
Thyroid examination, 283-285
Thyrotoxicosis, 702
Timed stands test, 666

Tinel sign, 628
Toes, 624, 625, 680
Tongue
  biting, in seizures, 265
  fissured, 263
  indentations on tip of, 276
  in myasthenia gravis, 273
  vitamin B complex deficiency and, 267, 272
  wrong-way deviation, 830
Tooth erosion
  in acid reflux disease, 274
  in bulimia, 791
  in cocaine users, 815, 816
Tophaceous deposition in finger pads, 637
Torture victims, 843, 848
Transforming growth factor, 177
Transvaginal sonography, pelvic examination vs., 36
Trapezius muscle weakness, 669
Traube's space, 510
Tremors, 676
Tricuspid regurgitation, 370, 371
Trident tongue, in myasthenia gravis, 273
Tuberculosis, 89, 774
Tumors, percussion in assessment of, 30
Two-point discrimination test, 782
Type A behavior, 418
Typhoid state, 104

U

Ulcers
  aphthous, 769
  foot, infected, 620
  ischemic, 446
  leg, 184
  peptic, 464, 707
Ulnar collateral flow, 438-440
Ultrasonography, 37; see also
    Echocardiography
  abdominal, 441, 444
  pelvic examination vs., 36
  prostate, 537
Unconsciousness, 793
Upper limb, 627-638
  abducted arm as sign of ruptured cervical disc, 665

About the Authors

Henry Schneiderman, MD, FACP, struggled with a deep attraction to classics. He graduated from Tufts University School of Medicine in 1976 and completed residencies in anatomic pathology and internal medicine. His later faculty-development training in geriatrics was under the joint aegis of the Travelers Center on Aging of the University of Connecticut, and the John A. Hartford Foundation. Presently he enjoys leading a "wonderfully skilled and humane group of geriatric clinician-teachers" at the nonsectarian, not-for-profit Hebrew Home & Hospital of West Hartford, Connecticut. Nonprofessional activity centers on his wife and their child. He reads literature and history, and confesses to writing poems.

Aldo Peixoto (Filho), MD, is the son of a physician from Florianopolis, Brazil, where he developed a deep interest in the kidney during his days at the University of Santa Caterina School of Medicine, from which he graduated in 1991. Upon completion of residency training with distinction at the University of Connecticut program, he served as an outstanding Chief Medical Resident. His superior interpersonal skills and consummate scholarship led to his being invited to co-author the present text at this early point in his career. He is currently completing a fellowship in nephrology at Yale University School of Medicine.

Parting Shot

Perhaps the reader will enjoy the perspective of one of our professional forebears on the subjects of this bibliography. Two centuries ago, the sometimes unmet need for bedside experience in the training of doctors was already well established. So was the intellectual honesty of looking to the diagnostic touchstone of autopsy:

> [The student] must Join Examples with Study, before he can be sufficiently qualified to prescribe for the sick, for Language and Books alone can never give him Adequate Ideals of Diseases and the best methods of treating them. [There is also a need for bedside teaching where] the Clinical professor comes to the Aid of Speculation and demonstrates the Truth of Theory by Facts. [There the professor] meets his pupils at stated times in the Hospital, and when a case presents adapted to his purpose, he asks all those Questions which lead to a certain knowledge of the Disease and parts Affected; and if the Disease baffles the power of the Art and the patient [dies], he then brings his Knowledge to the Test, and fixes honour or discredit on his Reputation by exposing all the Morbid parts to View, and Demonstrates by what means it produced Death, and if perchance he finds something unexpected, which Betrays an Error in Judgment, he like a great and good man immediately acknowledges the mistake, and, for the benefit of survivors, points out other methods by which it might have been more happily treated.

Thomas Bond, University of Pennsylvania, 1776